SOMATICS EXERCISES FOR WEIGHT LOSS

Healing from Mind to Body

Lucy Connor

In the quiet spaces of my life, where the daily hustle took a pause, I found myself standing at the crossroads of discomfort and curiosity. My body carried the weight of stress, both figuratively and literally. The sedentary demands of work, the relentless pace of life, and the silent battles with self-esteem manifested in the extra pounds that clung stubbornly.

It was in this moment of unease that I stumbled upon somatic exercises. Intrigued by the promise of mindful movement and the integration of body and mind, I tentatively began my somatic journey. What started as a series of gentle exercises soon transformed into a profound exploration of self.

The somatic approach unfolded like a revelation. The exercises weren't just about physical movement; they became gateways to understanding the intricate dialogues between my body and mind. As I tuned into the subtleties of my breath, the sensations of my muscles, and the whispers of my thoughts, a transformative process was set in motion.

Weight loss, while not the primary goal, became a natural outcome of this holistic practice. The exercises weren't punitive; they were an invitation to move joyfully, mindfully, and with a newfound respect for my body. It was not about shedding pounds but shedding the weight of self-judgment, embracing self-compassion, and understanding the rhythms of my body.

The more I delved into somatic exercises, the more I discovered the interconnectedness of physical and mental well-being. Stress, which had once manifested as tension in my muscles and excess weight, began to dissipate. The somatic practices became my sanctuary, a refuge where I could unwind, reset, and find a sense of calm amid life's storms.

Empowered by the changes I experienced, I felt compelled to share this transformative journey. It wasn't just about weight loss; it was about reclaiming a sense of self, fostering a mindful relationship with the body, and discovering the joy of movement. This book is born out of gratitude for the newfound vitality, the renewed sense of self, and the profound changes that somatic exercises brought into my life.

May these pages be a companion to others seeking a path to holistic well-being. May the somatic adventure be as transformative for you as it has been for me.

With gratitude,

Lucy Connor

Copyright © 2024 Lucy Connor

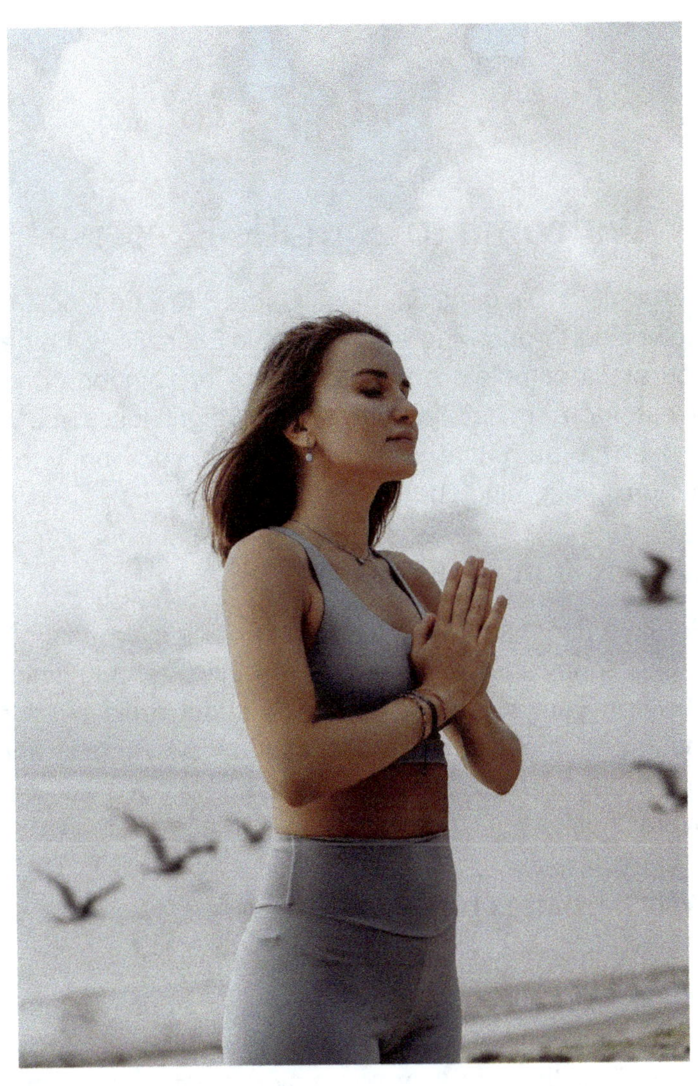

Introduction

Welcome to Somatic Exercise

Welcome to a transformative journey towards holistic well-being through the art of Somatic Exercise. Whether you are a complete novice to fitness or someone on a quest for a mindful approach to weight loss, you've chosen a path that not only shapes your body but nurtures your mind and spirit.

What is Somatic Exercise?

Somatic Exercise is not just a series of movements; it's a philosophy that understands the intimate connection between your mind and body. It's about rediscovering the joy of movement, fostering body awareness, and embracing the profound impact this can have on your overall health.

Why Somatics for Weight Loss?

Traditional approaches to weight loss often focus solely on external factors like caloric intake, rigorous workouts, and restrictive diets. Somatics takes a different path. It recognizes that the way you move, breathe, and carry stress in your body can significantly influence your weight.

In this book, we'll guide you through gentle yet powerful movements that not only sculpt your physique but also address the root causes of stress-related weight gain. We'll explore the connection between your emotional well-being and your body, offering you a holistic approach to sustainable weight management.

What to Expect in this Book:

1. **Foundations of Somatic Exercise:** Understand the principles that form the basis of somatic movement. Learn how simple yet mindful movements can be the key to unlocking a healthier, happier you.

2. **Getting Started:** We'll ease you into the practice, providing tips on setting up your space, focusing on breathwork, and cultivating the right mindset for your somatic journey.

3. **Somatics and Weight Loss:** Discover how stress impacts your weight and how somatic exercises can be a gentle yet effective antidote. This section is not just about shedding pounds; it's about embracing a lifestyle that supports your well-being.

4. **30-Day Somatic Exercise Challenge:** Ready for a transformative experience? We've designed a 30-day challenge to kickstart your somatic journey. Each day

brings you closer to a stronger, more mindful version of yourself.

5. **Daily Routines and Weekly Plans:** We'll help you integrate somatic exercises seamlessly into your daily life. From morning wake-ups to evening relaxation, these routines are designed to fit your schedule.

Your Journey Starts Now:

Embark on this journey with an open heart and a willingness to explore the capabilities of your body and mind. Throughout this book, we'll be your companions, offering guidance, support, and encouragement every step of the way.

The beauty of somatic exercise lies not just in the destination but in the journey itself. It's a journey of self-discovery, resilience, and transformation. Are you ready to embrace it?

Understanding the Mind–Body Connection

Embarking on your somatic exercise journey involves more than just physical movements; it's a profound exploration of the intricate dance between your mind and body. Let's delve into the essence of the mind-body connection and discover why it's at the heart of somatic exercise.

The Unity of Mind and Body:

In the realm of somatics, we embrace the fundamental truth that the mind and body are not separate entities but interconnected aspects of our being. Your thoughts, emotions, and experiences are not confined to your mind alone; they are imprinted in the way you carry tension, move, and hold yourself.

The Impact of Stress:

Consider stress as a prime example. When stress permeates your mind, your body responds, often tightening certain muscles or causing discomfort. Chronic stress can manifest in physical ailments, impacting everything from digestion to sleep. Conversely, the state of your body can influence your mental state, creating a continuous loop.

Somatics as a Mindful Practice:

Somatic exercise invites you to be present, to listen to the whispers of your body, and to understand the stories it tells. As you engage in these gentle movements, you're not just addressing physical tension; you're also unraveling the layers of stress stored in your muscles.

Breath as a Bridge:

Central to the mind-body connection is the breath, a bridge between the conscious and the subconscious. Mindful breathing anchors you in the present moment, creating a pathway to release physical and mental tension. In this book, we'll guide you in harnessing the power of your breath to enhance your somatic practice.

Emotions in Motion:

As you engage in somatic exercises, you may find emotions surfacing. This is a natural and welcomed aspect of the mind-body connection. Somatic movement provides a safe space to explore and release stored emotions, fostering not just physical flexibility but emotional resilience.

The Mindful Approach to Weight Loss:

Understanding the mind-body connection is pivotal to our approach to weight loss. Somatics is not about quick fixes or rigid diets; it's about cultivating a mindful relationship with your body. By addressing the emotional and physical aspects of weight management, you're laying the foundation for lasting change.

Your Mind-Body Adventure Begins:

As you progress through this book, keep in mind that every movement is an opportunity to deepen your understanding of yourself. The mind-body connection is not a concept to be grasped but an ongoing exploration, a conversation between the wisdom of your body and the consciousness of your mind.

Ready to embark on this mindful adventure? Let's proceed to practical exercises that will not only shape your body but also enrich your understanding of the beautiful union between your mind and body.

Why Somatics for Weight Loss?

Welcome to the core of our somatic journey, where we unravel the unique benefits that make somatic exercise an exceptional and holistic approach to weight loss. Let's explore why somatics goes beyond traditional methods and how it can be your key to sustainable and mindful weight management.

Mindful Movement, Sustainable Results:

In the world of weight loss, fad diets and intense workout routines often promise rapid results. Somatic exercise, however, takes a different path. It's not about pushing your body to its limits but about cultivating a mindful and sustainable approach to movement

Addressing Stress-Related Weight Gain:

Stress is a silent contributor to weight gain, and somatics understands this connection. When stress becomes chronic, it can lead to emotional eating, disrupted sleep, and an accumulation of visceral fat. Somatic exercises become a powerful tool to unwind the stress stored in your body, breaking the cycle of stress-related weight gain.

Release Tension, Release Weight:

The body often holds onto tension in the form of tight muscles and restricted movement. Somatic exercises are designed to release this tension, not only alleviating discomfort but also facilitating weight loss. As you move with awareness, you're not just burning calories; you're allowing your body to function optimally.

Mindful Eating Practices:

Somatics extends beyond the mat and into your daily life, especially your relationship with food. By cultivating mindfulness in your movements, you naturally extend this awareness to your eating habits. Somatic exercise becomes a guide to intuitive and mindful eating, a key component of sustainable weight management.

Balancing Hormones Naturally:

Somatic movements, especially those designed to reduce stress, contribute to hormonal balance. Cortisol, the stress hormone, is known to influence weight. By engaging in mindful movements, you regulate cortisol levels, creating an environment conducive to weight loss.

Lifestyle, Not a Quick Fix:

One of the core principles of somatics is the idea that movement is a way of life, not just a means to an end. Somatic exercises are not temporary solutions but an invitation to adopt a lifestyle that supports overall well-being. The weight loss you achieve becomes a natural outcome of a balanced and mindful existence.

Cultivating a Positive Body Image:

Somatics is not about conforming to societal ideals of beauty but about fostering a positive and loving relationship with your body. As you engage in these movements, you'll witness the transformative power of self-acceptance, a mindset that transcends numbers on a scale.

A Holistic Approach to Your Transformation:

In the chapters that follow, we'll guide you through movements, breathwork, and mindfulness practices that form the tapestry of somatic exercise. Each exercise is not just a step towards weight loss; it's a brick in the construction of a healthier, more vibrant you.

Are you ready to embrace a weight loss journey that goes beyond the surface and touches the core of your being? Let's dive into the transformative world of somatic exercise.

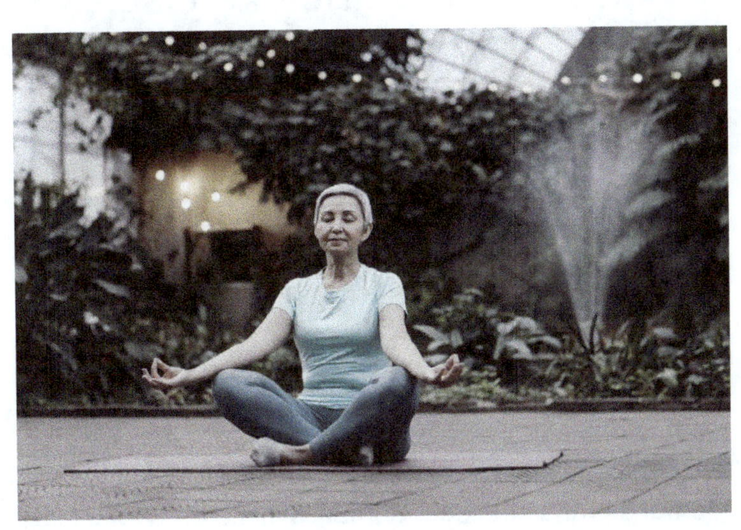

Chapter 1: Foundations of Somatic Exercise

What is Somatic Exercise?

Welcome to the heart of our somatic exploration, where we unravel the essence of somatic exercise and lay the groundwork for your transformative journey. Let's delve into the core principles that define somatics and understand why it's not just a set of movements but a philosophy that connects your mind, body, and spirit.

The Body as a Living Experience:

At the core of somatic exercise is the idea that your body is not just a machine to be trained; it's a dynamic, living experience. It's a vessel that stores your emotions, memories, and stresses. Somatics invites you to explore this living experience through intentional and mindful movements.

Mind-Body Connection:

Unlike traditional exercise that often focuses solely on physical outcomes, somatic exercise places a profound emphasis on the connection between your mind and body. It recognizes that the way you move reflects the state of your mind, and vice versa. Every movement becomes a conversation, an exploration of the intricate relationship between your conscious and subconscious self.

Sensory Awareness:

Central to somatic exercise is the cultivation of sensory awareness. It's about becoming attuned to the sensations within your body—the subtle tensions, the areas of ease, and the ever-present breath. Through this heightened awareness, you gain insight into the patterns that govern your movements and, by extension, your life.

Gentle Movements with Profound Impact:

Somatic exercises are characterized by their gentleness. They are not about pushing your body to extremes but about inviting it to move with intention and awareness. These gentle movements have a profound impact, releasing stored tension, improving flexibility, and fostering an overall sense of well-being.

Breath as the Bridge:

Your breath is not just a physiological function; it's the bridge between your conscious and subconscious realms. Somatic exercise places a significant focus on breathwork, using it as a tool to anchor your mind in the present moment, release tension, and deepen the mind-body connection.

Mindful Exploration, Not Repetition:

Unlike traditional exercises that often involve repetitive motions, somatic exercises encourage mindful exploration. Each movement is an opportunity to discover new facets of your body, to release habitual tensions, and to embrace a sense of curiosity and play in your physical practice.

A Journey, Not a Destination:

Somatic exercise is not a goal-oriented journey; it's a process, a continuous exploration of self. It's an invitation to move away from the mindset of achieving an external outcome and to immerse yourself in the richness of the present moment.

Ready to embark on this mindful journey through somatic exercise? Let's proceed to practical exercises that will not only shape your body but also enrich your understanding of the beautiful union between your mind and body.

Principles of Somatic Movement

As we delve into the world of somatic exercise, let's explore the guiding principles that shape this transformative practice. These principles are the compass for your journey offering direction, purpose, and a deep understanding of how somatics can be a profound agent of change in your life.

1. Mindful Awareness:

Somatic movement begins with awareness. It's about turning your attention inward, listening to the subtle signals your body communicates. Mindful awareness forms the cornerstone of somatic exercises, allowing you to observe, without judgment, the sensations, tensions, and movements within.

2. Sensory Perception:

Somatics is a sensory journey. It's about perceiving the nuances of movement, the gentle stretch of a muscle, the rhythm of your breath, the play of balance. Through heightened sensory perception, you'll cultivate a deeper connection with your body, unraveling its mysteries with each intentional movement.

3. Slow and Gentle Movements:

Unlike the rapid and forceful nature of some fitness routines, somatic movements are deliberate, slow, and gentle. This intentional pace allows you to engage with each movement fully, breaking away from the hurried pace of daily life and fostering a sense of tranquility in your practice.

4. Breath as a Guide:

Your breath is more than a physiological process; it's a guide in somatic movement. Connecting breath to movement not only enhances the efficiency of exercises but also serves as a bridge between the conscious and subconscious realms. Your breath becomes a steady companion on this mindful journey.

5. Curiosity and Exploration:

Somatic movement encourages curiosity and exploration. It's an invitation to approach each exercise with a sense of wonder, letting go of preconceived notions and embracing the potential for discovery. Through exploration, you'll uncover new pathways of movement and release.

6. Quality Over Quantity:

In somatic exercise, it's the quality of movement that takes precedence over quantity. It's not about how many repetitions you can perform but how deeply and consciously you can engage with each movement. This principle emphasizes precision and awareness over the sheer volume of exercises.

7. Release of Habitual Tension:

The body often accumulates tension due to habitual movements and stress. Somatic exercises are designed to release this tension. Through mindful movements, you'll gradually let go of patterns that no longer serve you, freeing your body to move with greater ease and flexibility.

8. Integration of Body and Mind:

Somatics is a holistic approach that acknowledges the inseparable connection between body and mind. Each movement is an opportunity to integrate these two aspects of yourself, creating a harmonious union that extends beyond the mat into your daily life.

As you embark on your somatic journey, keep these principles in mind. They are not just guidelines; they are the threads that weave the fabric of a transformative and mindful practice. Now, let's dive into practical exercises that embody these principles and set the stage for your somatic exploration.

Mindful Movement for Beginners

Embarking on your somatic journey begins with the simplicity of mindful movement. In this section, we'll gently introduce you to the foundational exercises that form the bedrock of somatic practice. These movements are not just about physicality; they are an invitation to cultivate awareness, explore your body, and begin your transformative journey.

1. Breath Awareness Exercise:

Begin by finding a comfortable seated or lying position. Close your eyes and bring your attention to your breath. Notice the inhales and exhales without altering them. Allow your breath to guide you into a state of relaxation. This exercise sets the stage for mindful awareness in all your movements.

2. Gentle Neck Rolls:

Sit or stand comfortably with your spine straight. Inhale as you gently tilt your head to one side, bringing your ear towards your shoulder. Exhale as you roll your head down and then inhale as you bring it up to the other side. These gentle neck rolls release tension and increase flexibility.

3. Shoulder Circles:

Stand or sit comfortably. Inhale as you lift your shoulders towards your ears, exhale as you roll them back and down. Repeat this motion, allowing your breath to guide the movement. This exercise promotes awareness of shoulder tension and encourages a release of stress.

4. Body Scan Meditation:

Lie down in a comfortable position. Close your eyes and bring your attention to each part of your body, starting from your toes and moving up to your head. Notice any areas of tension or discomfort. Breathe into these areas, allowing them to soften and release. This body scan meditation enhances your awareness of the body-mind connection.

5. Seated Forward Fold:

Sit comfortably with your legs extended in front of you. Inhale to lengthen your spine, and as you exhale, hinge at your hips and reach towards your toes. Let your hands rest wherever they comfortably reach. Focus on the sensations in your hamstrings and lower back. This forward fold encourages a mindful stretch.

6. Mindful Walking:

Take a slow walk, paying close attention to each step. Feel the connection of your foot with the ground, notice the shift of weight, and be present in the act of walking. Mindful walking brings awareness to the simple yet profound movement of each step.

7. Breath and Movement Coordination:

Incorporate your breath into simple movements. For example, inhale as you raise your arms, exhale as you lower them. Coordinate your breath with your movements, enhancing the mind-body connection.

8. Savasana (Corpse Pose):

Lie down on your back with legs extended and arms by your sides. Close your eyes and focus on your breath.

This relaxation pose allows you to integrate the benefits of your mindful movements and invites a deep sense of calm.

Remember, these are introductory exercises to initiate you into the world of somatic movement. As you engage with these movements, approach them with a sense of curiosity and openness. Your journey is unique, and these exercises are your first steps towards a more mindful and embodied way of moving through life. Let's now transition into the practical exercises that embody these principles and set the stage for your ongoing somatic exploration.

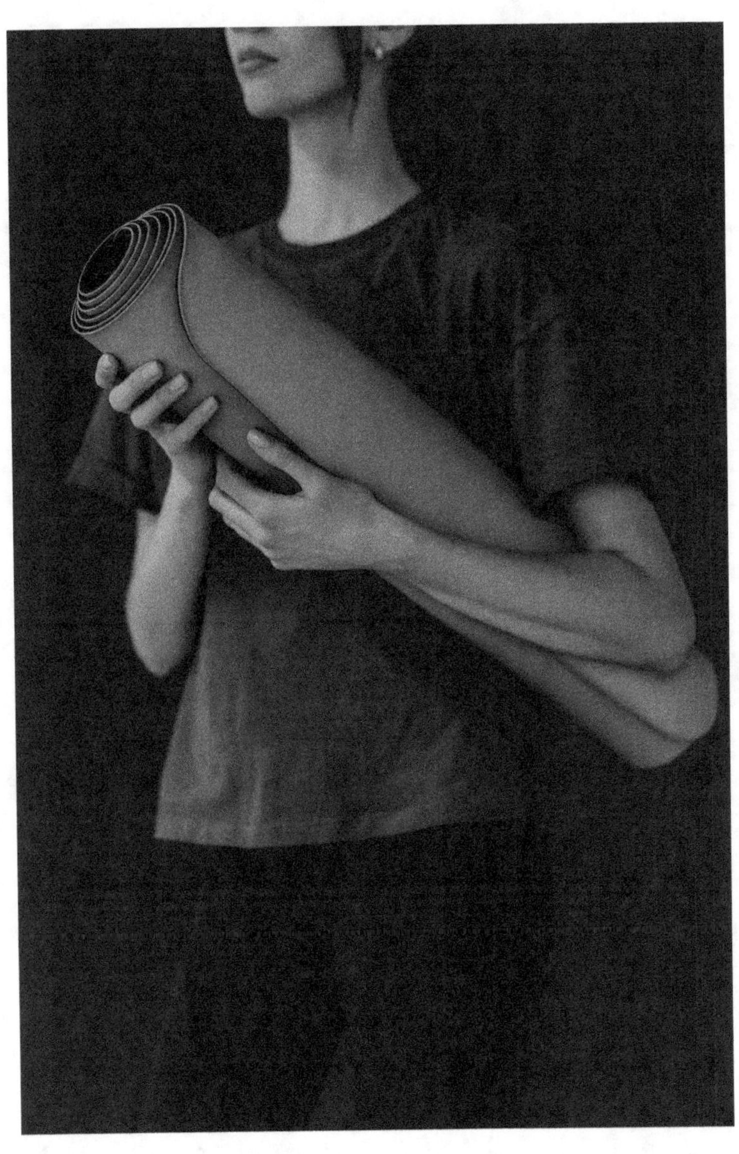

Chapter 2: Getting Started

Preparing Your Mind and Space

Before you embark on your somatic journey, take a moment to prepare your mind and create a space that nurtures mindfulness and exploration. This section guides you through the steps to set the stage for a positive and transformative experience.

1. Cultivate a Mindful Mindset:

Somatic exercise is not just about physical movement; it's a practice of mindfulness. Before you begin, find a quiet moment to sit comfortably and bring your awareness to the present. Take a few deep breaths, letting go of any mental clutter. Cultivate an open and curious mindset, free from expectations.

2. Set an Intention:

Consider setting an intention for your somatic practice. What aspect of yourself or your well-being would you like to nurture? Whether it's releasing tension, improving flexibility, or simply fostering a sense of calm, having a clear intention adds purpose to your practice.

3. Create a Dedicated Space:

Find a quiet and clutter-free space where you can move freely. It doesn't need to be large; even a corner of a room will suffice. Remove any distractions and create an environment that invites tranquility. Consider dimming the lights or using soft lighting to enhance the calming atmosphere.

4. Gather Essential Props:

You may want to have a few props nearby, such as a yoga mat, a cushion for seated exercises, or a blanket for warmth during relaxation. Having these items within reach ensures that you can fully immerse yourself in the practice without interruptions.

5. Turn Off Distractions:

Silence your phone or set it to "Do Not Disturb" mode. Consider playing soft instrumental music or nature sounds if it enhances your focus. The goal is to create a space where you can fully engage with the subtle sensations of your body without external disruptions.

6. Dress Comfortably:

Choose clothing that allows for unrestricted movement. Comfort is key in somatic exercise, and wearing loose, breathable attire ensures that your body can move freely without any restrictions.

7. Mindful Posture Check:

Before you start, take a moment to check your posture. Whether you're sitting or standing, ensure that your spine is aligned and your shoulders are relaxed. This mindful posture check establishes a foundation for awareness in movement.

8. Breath Awareness:

Bring attention to your breath. Take a few deep, intentional breaths to center yourself. Notice the natural rhythm of your breath, and let it guide you into the present moment. Your breath is a constant companion throughout your somatic practice.

9. Express Gratitude:

Before you begin your movements, take a moment to express gratitude. Gratitude for the opportunity to engage in mindful movement, for the capabilities of your body, and for the time you've dedicated to your well-being.

Now that you've prepared your mind and space, you're ready to embark on your somatic journey. Let's transition into the practical exercises that embody these principles and invite you into the transformative world of somatic movement.

The Importance of Breath in Somatics

As you step into the realm of somatic exercises, understand that your breath is not just a biological function; it's a guiding force that intertwines with every movement. In this section, we delve into the profound significance of breath in somatics and how it becomes a catalyst for a mindful and transformative practice.

1. Breath as the Bridge:

Your breath serves as a bridge between the conscious and subconscious realms. In somatic exercises, it acts as a constant companion, linking your awareness to the present moment. With each inhale and exhale, you're invited to synchronize your movements, creating a dance between breath and body.

2. Facilitating Mind-Body Connection:

Conscious breathing facilitates a deeper connection between your mind and body. As you engage in somatic movements with an awareness of your breath, you begin to unravel the intricate dialogue between physical sensations, emotions, and thoughts. Breath becomes a unifying force that integrates your entire being.

3. Enhancing Mindfulness:

Mindfulness is at the core of somatic practice, and your breath is a primary vehicle for cultivating this awareness. The rhythmic flow of your breath becomes an anchor, grounding you in the present moment and allowing you to fully immerse yourself in each movement.

4. Release of Tension:

Breath is intimately linked to the release of tension. In somatics, as you consciously breathe into areas of tension, you signal to your body that it's safe to let go. The gentle exhale becomes a vehicle for releasing stored stress, allowing muscles to soften and promoting a sense of relaxation.

5. Energetic Flow:

Consider your breath as a carrier of vital energy. In somatic exercises, each breath infuses your movements with a flow of energy, creating a sense of vitality and aliveness. As you move with the breath, you tap into a reservoir of inner strength and resilience.

6. Conscious Control and Precision:

Somatic movements are not just about the physicality of the motion; they are about the precision and conscious control that breath brings. The breath guides the pace of your movements, ensuring that each gesture is intentional and aligned with the rhythm of your breath.

7. Centering and Grounding:

Your breath is a tool for centering and grounding. In moments of complexity or challenge, returning to the breath becomes an anchor. The steady inhales and exhales provide a focal point, allowing you to navigate the intricacies of each movement with a sense of stability.

8. Cultivating Presence:

Through breath, you cultivate a heightened sense of presence. As you breathe into each moment, you're less likely to be carried away by distractions or intrusive thoughts. The breath becomes a guide, inviting you to fully inhabit the richness of your somatic experience.

In somatic exercises, your breath is not a passive component; it's an active and transformative force. As you engage in the practical exercises that follow, let your breath be your guide, a steady companion on your journey to greater self-awareness and well-being.

Proper Posture and Alignment

As you embark on your somatic journey, understanding and maintaining proper posture and alignment is fundamental. This section guides you through the key principles, ensuring that your movements are not only effective but also safe and supportive of your overall well-being.

1. Spinal Alignment:

Begin by establishing a neutral spine. Whether you're sitting, standing, or lying down, imagine a straight line extending from the base of your spine to the top of your head. Aligning your spine properly forms the foundation for all somatic movements, allowing for optimal energy flow and muscular engagement.

2. Head and Neck Position:

Ensure that your head is aligned with your spine. It shouldn't jut forward or droop down. Imagine a string gently lifting the crown of your head towards the ceiling. This alignment not only prevents strain on your neck but also promotes a sense of openness and ease.

3. Shoulder Placement:

Relax your shoulders and let them naturally fall away from your ears. Engaging in somatic exercises with relaxed shoulders prevents unnecessary tension and promotes a more fluid range of motion. Be mindful of any creeping tension, especially during movements that involve the upper body.

4. Hip Alignment:

For both standing and seated exercises, align your hips with your spine. Sit or stand with your weight evenly distributed between both hips. This balanced alignment ensures that your movements originate from your center, fostering stability and preventing undue stress on one side.

5. Knee and Ankle Alignment:

In weight-bearing exercises, such as lunges or squats, be mindful of your knee and ankle alignment. Your knees should be in line with your toes, not collapsing inward or splaying outward. This alignment supports the integrity of your joints and prevents unnecessary strain.

6. Engaging the Core:

Activate your core muscles gently but consistently. Your core, including the muscles around your abdomen and lower back, plays a pivotal role in maintaining stability. Engaging the core not only supports your spine but also enhances the efficacy of your movements.

7. Balanced Weight Distribution:

Whether you're standing or sitting, distribute your body weight evenly. Avoid favoring one side over the other. This balanced weight distribution promotes symmetry in your movements and prevents the development of muscle imbalances.

8. Mindful Body Scan:

Before each somatic exercise, conduct a quick body scan. Start from your head and move down to your toes, checking for any areas of tension or misalignment. This mindful body scan helps you tune into your body and make subtle adjustments for optimal posture.

9. Comfortable Positioning:

Lastly, ensure that you are in a comfortable position for each exercise. Whether sitting, standing, or lying down, your comfort contributes to your ability to fully engage with the movements without distraction.

By prioritizing proper posture and alignment, you're not only optimizing the effectiveness of your somatic practice but also nurturing the health of your body. As you move forward into the practical exercises, keep these principles in mind, making adjustments as needed to maintain a posture that supports your well-being.

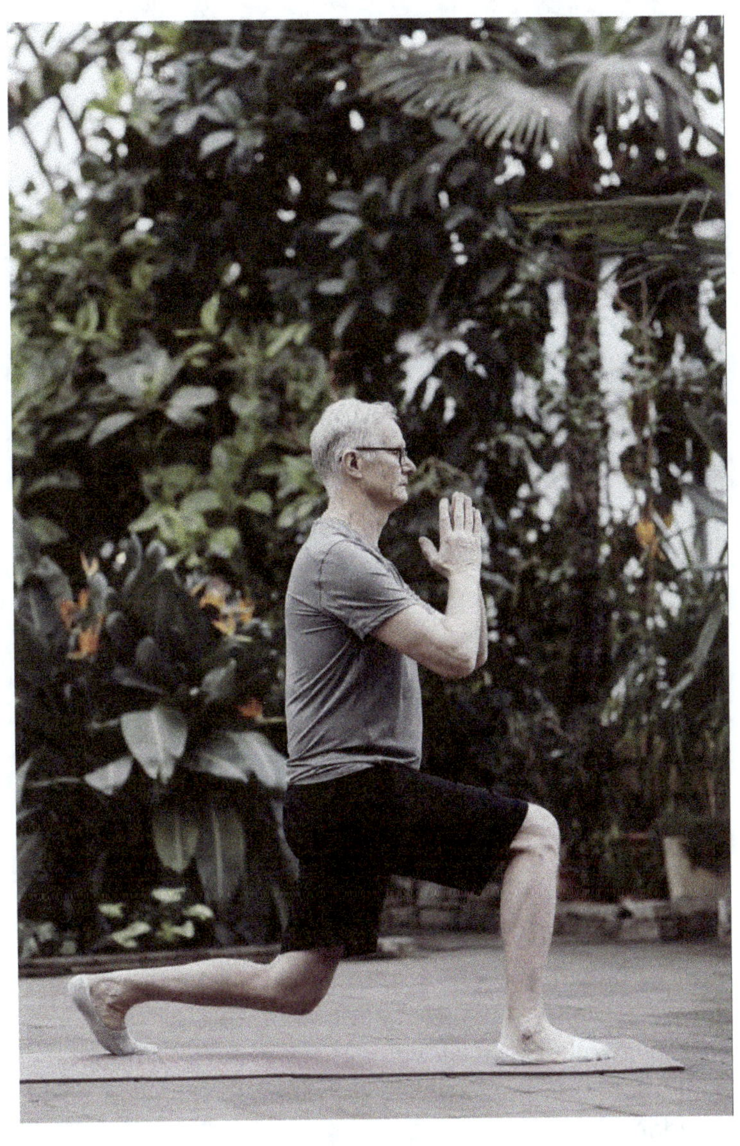

Chapter 3: Exploring Somatic Exercises

Gentle Warm-Up Movements

Before you dive into the deeper somatic exercises, it's crucial to gently awaken your body. The following warm-up movements are designed to increase blood flow, improve flexibility, and enhance your mind-body connection. Take your time with each movement, and let your breath guide you into a state of readiness.

1. Neck Rolls:

Start by sitting or standing comfortably. Inhale as you gently tilt your head to one side, bringing your ear towards your shoulder. Exhale as you roll your head down and then inhale as you bring it up to the other side. Repeat this motion for about 1 minute, letting go of any tension in your neck.

2. Shoulder Rolls:

Stand with your feet hip-width apart. Inhale as you lift your shoulders towards your ears, exhale as you roll them back and down. Repeat this motion, allowing your breath to guide the movement. Continue for about 1-2 minutes, focusing on releasing tension in your shoulders.

3. Gentle Arm Swings:

Stand with your feet shoulder-width apart. Extend your arms out to the sides. Inhale as you swing your arms forward, and exhale as you swing them back. Let the movement originate from your shoulders. Repeat for about 1-2 minutes, allowing your breath to sync with the swinging motion.

4. Spinal Twist:

Sit or stand with your spine straight. Inhale as you lengthen your spine, and exhale as you twist gently to one side. Inhale back to the center, and exhale as you twist to the other side. Repeat for about 1-2 minutes, feeling the gentle stretch along your spine.

5. Hip Circles:

Stand with your feet hip-width apart. Inhale as you circle your hips clockwise, and exhale as you circle them counterclockwise. Continue for about 1-2 minutes, allowing your breath to guide the circular motion and promoting flexibility in your hip joints.

6. Knee Lifts:

Stand with your feet hip-width apart. Inhale as you lift one knee towards your chest, and exhale as you lower it back down. Repeat with the other knee. Continue alternating for about 1-2 minutes, maintaining a steady and controlled pace.

7. Ankle Rolls:

Sit or stand comfortably. Lift one foot off the ground and gently roll your ankle clockwise, then counterclockwise. Repeat with the other foot. Continue for about 1 minute, paying attention to any areas of stiffness and encouraging flexibility in your ankles.

8. Full Body Shake:

Stand with your feet shoulder-width apart. Inhale deeply, and as you exhale, shake your entire body starting from your hands and gradually moving down to your feet. Let go of any tension, and continue shaking for about 1-2 minutes, allowing your body to release accumulated stress.

Remember, the key to a successful warm-up is to move gently and with awareness. These movements are not about intensity; they're about preparing your body for the mindful journey ahead. As you complete the warm-up, transition seamlessly into the upcoming somatic exercises with a body that is ready and receptive.

Basic Somatic Movements for Beginners

Welcome to the core of your somatic journey. These basic movements are designed for beginners, offering a gentle introduction to the principles of somatic exercise. Approach each movement with mindfulness and curiosity, and let your breath guide you as you explore the nuances of your body.

1. Pelvic Tilt:

Purpose: Release tension in the lower back and hips.

- Lie on your back with your knees bent and feet hip-width apart.
- Inhale as you tilt your pelvis forward, arching your lower back slightly.
- Exhale as you tilt your pelvis backward, flattening your lower back against the mat.
- Repeat this gentle rocking motion for about 1-2 minutes, coordinating with your breath.

2. Shoulder Circles:

Purpose: Relieve tension in the shoulders and upper back.

- Stand or sit comfortably with your spine straight.
- Inhale as you lift your shoulders towards your ears.
- Exhale as you roll your shoulders back and down.

- Repeat this circular motion for about 1-2 minutes, allowing your breath to guide the movement.

3. Cat–Cow Stretch:

Purpose: Increase flexibility and awareness in the spine.

- Start on your hands and knees in a tabletop position.
- Inhale as you arch your back, dropping your belly towards the floor (Cow Pose).
- Exhale as you round your back, tucking your chin to your chest (Cat Pose).
- Repeat this flowing movement for about 1-2 minutes, syncing your breath with the motion.

4. Seated Forward Fold:

Purpose: Stretch the muscles of the lower back and hamstrings.

- Sit with your legs extended in front of you.
- Inhale to lengthen your spine.
- Exhale as you hinge at your hips and reach towards your toes.
- Hold for a few breaths, feeling a gentle stretch along your back and hamstrings.
- Repeat for about 1-2 minutes, allowing your breath to guide your movements.

5. Leg Lifts:

Purpose: Strengthen and engage the core muscles.

- Lie on your back with your legs extended.
- Inhale as you lift one leg towards the ceiling.
- Exhale as you lower the leg back down without touching the floor.
- Repeat with the other leg.
- Continue alternating for about 1-2 minutes, coordinating with your breath.

6. Side Bend Stretch:

Purpose: Increase flexibility and release tension in the sides of the body.

- Stand with your feet hip-width apart.
- Inhale as you reach one arm overhead, leaning gently to the side.
- Exhale as you return to the center.
- Repeat on the other side.
- Continue this side-to-side movement for about 1-2 minutes, allowing your breath to guide the stretch.

7. Hip Flexor Stretch:

Purpose: Stretch and release tension in the hip flexors.

- Kneel on your right knee with your left foot in front, forming a 90-degree angle.

- Inhale as you gently shift your weight forward, feeling a stretch in the right hip.
- Exhale as you return to the starting position.
- Repeat on the other side.
- Continue this alternating stretch for about 1-2 minutes, syncing with your breath.

8. Body Scan Meditation:

Purpose: Cultivate mindfulness and awareness of your body.

- Sit or lie down in a comfortable position.
- Close your eyes and bring your attention to different parts of your body, starting from your toes and moving up to your head.
- Inhale as you focus on an area, and exhale as you release any tension.
- Continue this mindful body scan for about 2-3 minutes, breathing into each part of your body.

Remember, these basic movements are the building blocks of your somatic practice. Take your time, move with intention, and let each breath guide you into a deeper connection with your body. As you progress, these movements will serve as a solid foundation for more advanced somatic exercises. Enjoy the journey!

Introduction to Body Scanning

Welcome to the practice of body scanning, an invaluable tool in your somatic journey. Body scanning is a mindfulness technique that involves directing your attention to different parts of your body, fostering awareness, and creating a profound connection between your mind and body. As we explore this practice, let curiosity be your guide, and let your breath be the gentle companion that accompanies you through each scan.

1. Understanding Body Scanning:

Purpose: To cultivate awareness and presence in each part of the body.

Body scanning is a practice of systematically directing your attention to various regions of your body, observing sensations, tensions, or areas of ease. It is a journey of self-discovery, allowing you to tune into the subtle signals that your body communicates.

2. The Power of Mindful Attention:

Purpose: To harness the transformative potential of focused awareness.

Our bodies are often overlooked in the hustle and bustle of daily life. Through body scanning, you bring a spotlight of attention to each part, fostering a mindful presence that is often absent. This intentional focus opens the door to a deeper understanding of your body's unique language.

3. Benefits of Body Scanning:

- **Stress Reduction:** By systematically scanning and releasing tension, body scanning can be a powerful stress reduction technique.
- **Improved Body Awareness:** Regular practice enhances your ability to detect subtle sensations and changes within your body.
- **Emotional Connection:** Body scanning provides a pathway to connect with and process emotions stored in different areas of the body.

4. Preparing for Body Scanning:

- Find a quiet and comfortable space where you won't be disturbed.
- Sit or lie down in a relaxed position.
- Close your eyes to enhance your inward focus.
- Take a few deep breaths to center yourself.

5. The Body Scan Process:

- Begin with your toes and gradually move up through your body or vice versa.
- As you direct your attention to each area, notice any sensations without judgment.
- If you encounter tension, gently breathe into that area and allow it to soften.

- Spend a few breaths on each part before moving on.

6. Cultivating a Gentle Awareness:

- Approach each part of the body with a sense of curiosity and openness.
- Let go of expectations or judgments.
- Your goal is not to change anything but to observe and be present with whatever arises.

7. Using Breath as a Guide:

- Your breath is the thread that weaves through the tapestry of the body scan.
- Use the breath to anchor your awareness, syncing it with the rhythm of your scan.
- Inhale into the area you're focusing on, and exhale any tension or discomfort.

8. Closing the Body Scan:

- Once you've scanned your entire body, take a few moments to bask in the awareness you've cultivated.
- Gently bring your attention back to your breath and the present moment.
- When you're ready, open your eyes if they were closed.

Body scanning is not a task; it's an invitation to be present with yourself. As you integrate this practice into your somatic routine, you'll discover the richness that lies within each part of your body. Now, let's transition into practical exercises where body scanning becomes a cornerstone of your somatic exploration.

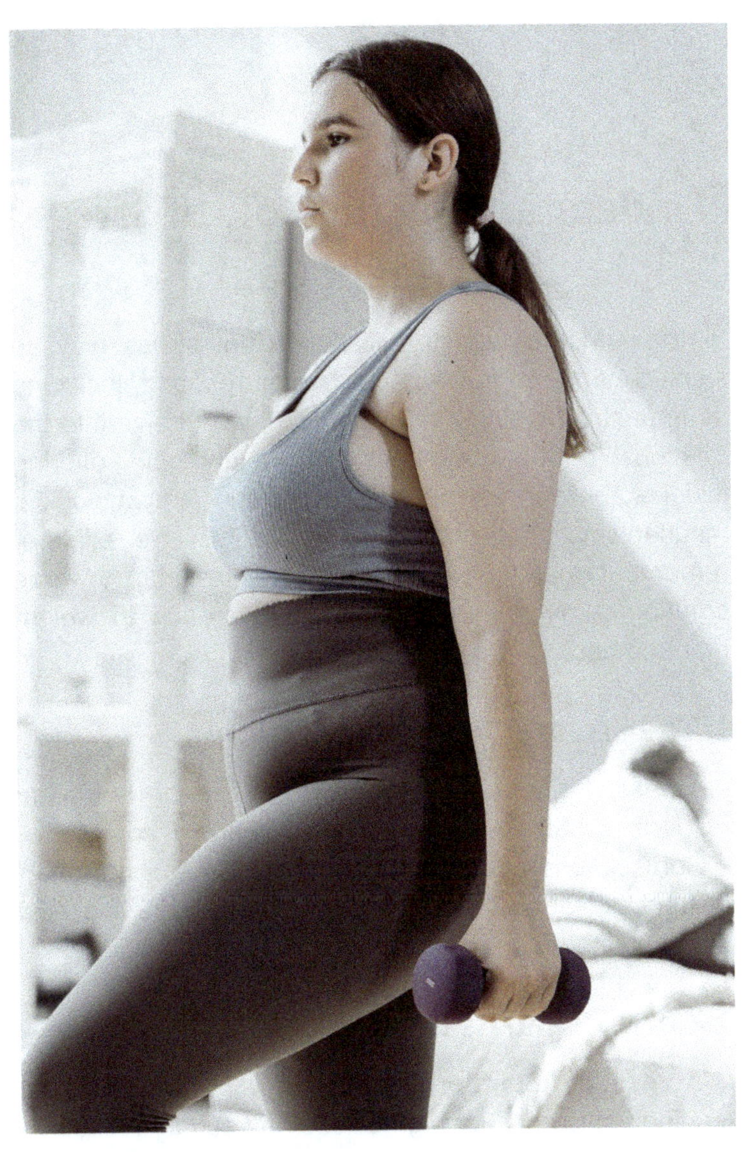

Chapter 4: Somatics and Weight Loss

Understanding the Role of Stress in Weight Gain

In the intricate tapestry of well-being, stress plays a significant role in the way our bodies respond, including its impact on weight. In this section, we'll delve into the relationship between stress and weight gain, offering insights into the physiological and psychological mechanisms that connect the two. As we explore, remember that this knowledge is a key step towards creating a mindful and balanced approach to weight management.

1. The Stress-Weight Connection:

- Stress triggers a complex interplay of hormonal responses in the body, notably the release of cortisol.
- Cortisol, often referred to as the "stress hormone," influences various metabolic processes, including how the body stores and uses energy.

2. Cortisol and its Impact:

- **Increased Appetite:** Cortisol can stimulate appetite, leading to cravings for high-calorie and sugary foods.

- **Fat Storage:** Chronic stress is associated with the accumulation of visceral fat, particularly around the abdominal area.

3. Emotional Eating and Coping Mechanisms:

- Stress can trigger emotional eating as a coping mechanism.
- Consuming comfort foods, often high in sugars and fats, can provide temporary relief from stress but may contribute to weight gain in the long run.

4. Impact on Metabolism:

- Prolonged stress can influence metabolic rate, potentially slowing it down.
- Reduced metabolism can make it more challenging to maintain or lose weight.

5. Disruption of Sleep Patterns:

- Stress can disrupt sleep patterns, leading to inadequate or poor-quality sleep.
- Sleep deprivation is linked to hormonal imbalances that can contribute to weight gain.

6. Chronic Inflammation:

- Persistent stress can contribute to chronic inflammation, which is associated with various health issues, including weight-related concerns.

- Chronic inflammation may interfere with the body's ability to regulate weight effectively.

7. Mind-Body Connection:

- Stress isn't solely a physical response; it also influences our mindset and behavior.
- Chronic stress can lead to a negative impact on self-care practices, including exercise and mindful eating.

8. Breaking the Stress-Weight Cycle:

- **Mindfulness Practices:** Incorporate mindfulness techniques such as meditation and deep breathing to manage stress.
- **Regular Physical Activity:** Engage in regular exercise to counteract the physiological effects of stress.
- **Healthy Coping Strategies:** Identify and adopt healthy coping mechanisms that don't involve emotional eating.

9. Holistic Well-being:

- Recognizing and addressing stress is a pivotal part of a holistic approach to well-being.
- Combining stress management strategies with a balanced diet and regular exercise forms a comprehensive strategy for weight management.

Understanding the relationship between stress and weight gain empowers you to make informed choices that contribute to both physical and mental health. As you progress through this book, consider it not just as a guide to physical exercises but as a holistic approach to well-being, addressing stress as a crucial factor in your weight management journey.

Somatics for Stress Reduction

In the fast-paced rhythm of modern life, stress can accumulate in both body and mind. Somatic exercises offer a unique and effective approach to release tension, promote relaxation, and restore balance. Let's explore how somatic practices can be your sanctuary amidst life's demands, providing a pathway to a calmer and more centered existence.

1. Mindful Breath as the Anchor:

- Begin each somatic session with mindful breath awareness.
- Conscious breathing serves as an anchor, grounding you in the present moment and creating a foundation for stress reduction.

2. Gentle Body Scans:

- Practice body scans, systematically directing your attention to different parts of your body.
- Notice areas of tension or discomfort without judgment, and use your breath to release and soften those areas.

3. Slow and Fluid Movements

- Embrace slow and deliberate movements in your somatic exercises.
- Slowing down the pace allows you to fully experience each movement, fostering a sense of presence and reducing the rush of stress.

4. Release of Tension in Targeted Areas:

- Identify areas of your body where you commonly hold tension (e.g., shoulders, neck, jaw).
- Incorporate specific somatic exercises that target these areas, promoting release and relaxation.

5. Somatic Yoga Nidra for Deep Relaxation:

- Integrate somatic variations of Yoga Nidra, a practice known for deep relaxation.
- Through guided imagery and body awareness, you can release mental and physical tension, promoting a state of calmness.

6. Dynamic Stretching to Release Built-Up Energy:

- Engage in dynamic stretching, allowing your body to release built-up energy.
- Incorporate movements that involve a gentle stretch and release, providing a physical outlet for stress.

7. Grounding Techniques:

- Integrate grounding techniques into your somatic practice.
- Imagery, such as connecting with the support of the earth, can foster a sense of stability and calmness.

8. Progressive Relaxation Techniques:

- Practice progressive relaxation, systematically tensing and then releasing different muscle groups.
- This technique promotes a profound release of physical tension and can be seamlessly incorporated into somatic exercises.

9. Somatic Breathing Practices:

- Explore somatic breathing practices, such as diaphragmatic breathing.
- Engaging the diaphragm promotes relaxation by activating the body's parasympathetic nervous system.

10. Reflective Practices:

- End your somatic sessions with a few moments of reflection.
- Observe any shifts in your body, mind, or emotions, acknowledging the impact of the practice on your stress levels.

Somatics for stress reduction is not just a series of exercises; it's a holistic approach to well-being. As you engage in these practices, be present, be gentle with yourself, and let the somatic experience become a sanctuary where stress dissipates, and a tranquil calmness takes its place.

How Somatics Supports Healthy Weight Management

Embarking on a journey of healthy weight management involves more than just physical exercises and dietary changes. Somatics, with its unique focus on the mind-body connection, adds a profound dimension to your approach. In this section, we'll explore how somatics becomes a valuable ally in your quest for a balanced and healthy weight.

1. Mindful Eating Practices:

- Somatics encourages mindfulness in all aspects of life, including eating.
- Paying attention to the sensory experience of eating can foster healthier food choices and better digestion.

2. Stress Reduction and Weight:

- Chronic stress is often linked to weight gain.
- Somatic exercises, with their emphasis on relaxation and stress reduction, can help mitigate the impact of stress on your weight.

3. Body Awareness and Signals:

- Somatic practices enhance body awareness, helping you recognize hunger and fullness cues more effectively.
- Tuning into these signals allows for a more intuitive and mindful approach to eating.

4. Release of Emotional Tension:

- Emotional eating is a common challenge in weight management.
- Somatic exercises provide a means to release emotional tension, reducing the likelihood of turning to food for comfort.

5. Balanced Muscle Engagement:

- Somatic movements often focus on rebalancing muscle engagement and correcting posture.
- This balanced approach can contribute to a more efficient metabolism and improved body composition.

6. Enhanced Flexibility and Mobility:

- Improved flexibility and mobility, key outcomes of somatic exercises, support a more active lifestyle.
- Increased activity levels contribute to overall calorie expenditure and weight management.

7. Mind-Body Connection in Exercise:

- Somatic exercises emphasize the mind-body connection during movement.
- This awareness enhances the effectiveness of your workouts, ensuring that each movement is purposeful and aligned with your body's needs.

8. Reduced Joint and Muscle Pain:

- Chronic pain can limit physical activity, impacting weight management.
- Somatic practices alleviate tension and pain, creating an environment where regular exercise becomes more accessible.

9. Improved Posture and Core Strength:

- Somatic exercises often target the core muscles and posture.
- A strong core and good posture contribute to a more balanced physique and support overall physical well-being.

10. Cultivating a Positive Body Image:

- Somatic practices foster a positive relationship with your body.
- Embracing your body with acceptance and gratitude can positively influence your approach to healthy weight management.

Somatics is not just a series of movements; it's a holistic approach that aligns your mind and body to achieve well-being. As you integrate somatic practices into your routine, observe how they harmonize with your broader goals of healthy weight management. Let this journey be a celebration of the unity between your physical and mental well-being.

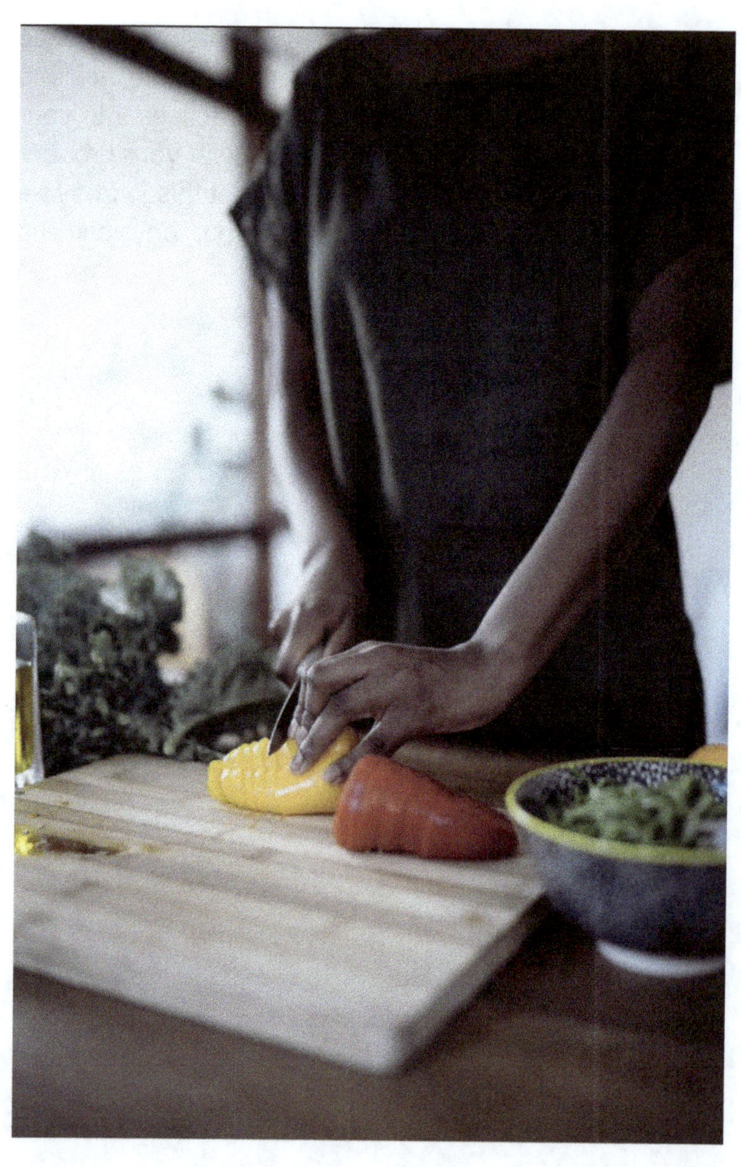

Chapter 5: Mindful Eating Practices

Mindful Eating and Somatic Awareness

Eating is not merely a physical act but an opportunity for a mindful connection with our bodies and the nourishment they receive. Combining the principles of mindful eating with somatic awareness creates a powerful synergy that transforms the way we approach and experience meals. Let's delve into how these practices can be seamlessly integrated into your daily life.

1. The Art of Mindful Eating:

- Mindful eating is the practice of paying full attention to the experience of eating without judgment.
- Engage all your senses in the act of eating, savoring the colors, textures, and flavors of your food.

2. Starting with Somatic Awareness:

- Before you begin eating, practice a brief somatic awareness exercise.
- Close your eyes, take a few deep breaths, and bring your attention to your body. Notice any areas of tension or relaxation.

3. Engaging the Breath:

- As you sit down to eat, take a moment to focus on your breath.
- Inhale deeply, exhale fully, allowing your breath to ground you in the present moment.

4. Savoring Each Bite:

- Take small, mindful bites, paying attention to the sensations in your mouth.
- Notice the flavors, textures, and how your body responds to each bite.

5. Listening to Hunger Cues:

- Use somatic awareness to tune into your body's hunger and fullness cues.
- Before reaching for seconds, check in with your body to see if you're genuinely hungry.

6. Releasing Tension During Meals:

- If you notice tension building up during a meal, pause.
- Engage in a brief somatic exercise, such as shoulder rolls or deep breathing, to release tension.

7. Mindful Presence, Not Multitasking:

- Avoid multitasking during meals.
- Eating with full attention allows you to savor the experience and recognize when you're satisfied.

8. Gratitude for Nourishment:

- Cultivate a sense of gratitude for the nourishment your meal provides.
- Reflect on the journey of the food from its source to your plate.

9. Mindful Snacking with Somatic Awareness:

- Extend mindful eating to snacks.
- Before grabbing a snack, pause, and engage in a brief somatic check-in.

10. Closing the Meal Mindfully:

- Conclude your meal with a moment of gratitude.
- Express thanks for the nourishment you've received and the opportunity to connect with your body.

Mindful eating and somatic awareness are not restrictive practices but rather invitations to savor and celebrate the act of nourishing your body. As you infuse these principles into your daily meals, observe the subtle transformations in your relationship with food and the deepening connection with your body. Let each bite be a celebration of mindfulness and self-awareness.

Connecting with Your Body's Hunger Signals

In the symphony of mindful eating, tuning into your body's hunger signals is akin to listening to the subtle notes that guide your nourishment. Let's explore the art of recognizing and responding to your body's cues, fostering a deeper connection with your innate wisdom and the sustenance it craves.

1. Understanding Hunger as a Spectrum:

- Hunger is not a binary state; it exists on a spectrum.
- Learn to recognize the different degrees of hunger, from a gentle rumble to a more pronounced sensation.

2. The Importance of Mindful Observation:

- Cultivate a habit of mindful observation of your body's signals.
- Regularly check in with yourself to identify where you fall on the hunger spectrum.

3. Physical vs. Emotional Hunger:

- Distinguish between physical hunger and emotional hunger.
- Physical hunger arises gradually and is located in the stomach, while emotional hunger tends to be sudden and is often tied to specific emotions.

4. Engaging the Senses:

- When hunger arises, engage your senses.
- Take a moment to notice the smells, sights, and anticipation of the food you're about to eat.

5. Checking In Before Meals:

- Before each meal, pause and check in with your body.
- Ask yourself how hungry you truly are and what type of food your body is craving.

6. Listening to Your Stomach:

- During meals, pay attention to your stomach.
- Eat slowly and pause to assess your level of fullness.

7. Honor Your Cravings Mindfully:

- Allow yourself to honor cravings mindfully.
- If you're craving a specific food, acknowledge it and enjoy it in moderation.

8. Hydration and Hunger:

- Sometimes, thirst can be mistaken for hunger.
- Stay hydrated and listen to your body to discern whether you're truly hungry or need fluids.

9. Mindful Snacking:

- Approach snacks with mindfulness.

- When snacking, check in with your body to ensure you're eating out of hunger rather than habit or boredom.

10. Reflecting After Meals:

- After meals, reflect on your eating experience.
- Were you satisfied? Did you eat mindfully? Use these reflections to guide future eating habits.

Connecting with your body's hunger signals is a journey of self-discovery. As you deepen this connection, you'll find that your body is a wise guide, leading you to nourishment that aligns with your true needs. Embrace the subtle dance between hunger and satisfaction, and let each mindful bite be a celebration of your body's innate wisdom.

Somatic Techniques for Healthy Eating Habits

In the realm of nourishment, somatic techniques offer a gateway to mindful and intentional eating. Let's explore how incorporating somatic practices can transform your relationship with food, paving the way for healthier eating habits and a harmonious connection between mind and body.

1. Body Scans Before Meals:

- Prior to meals, engage in a brief body scan.
- Notice any areas of tension and release them through gentle breaths, bringing a sense of calm to your body.

2. Breath Awareness at the Table:

- Practice breath awareness while sitting at the table.
- Take a few deep breaths before starting your meal to center yourself and bring a mindful presence to the act of eating.

3. Somatic Relaxation Techniques:

- Incorporate somatic relaxation techniques into your pre-meal routine.
- Techniques such as progressive muscle relaxation can help release tension, creating a relaxed environment for eating.

4. Mindful Chewing and Savoring:

- Consciously chew your food with awareness.
- Savor each bite, paying attention to the flavors and textures. Engage your senses fully.

5. Body-Centered Food Choices:

- Use somatic awareness to guide food choices.
- Before deciding what to eat, check in with your body to discern its preferences and nutritional needs.

6. Listening to Fullness Signals:

- While eating, periodically pause to check in with your body.
- Listen for signals of fullness, and honor them by slowing down or stopping when satisfied.

7. Mindful Eating Postures:

- Be mindful of your posture while eating.
- Sit comfortably, and maintain an upright posture to support optimal digestion and somatic awareness.

8. Gratitude for Nourishment:

- Cultivate a sense of gratitude for the food on your plate.
- Take a moment before eating to express thanks for the nourishment your meal provides.

9. Somatic Reflection After Meals:

- After meals, engage in a somatic reflection.
- Notice how your body feels, any changes in energy levels, and reflect on the overall experience of the meal.

10. Breath and Digestion:

- Conclude your meals with a few deep breaths.
- This practice supports digestion and transitions your body into a state of relaxation.

Somatic techniques weave a thread of awareness into the fabric of your eating habits, transforming meals into mindful rituals. As you embrace these practices, observe the profound shifts in how you relate to food, finding joy and nourishment in each bite. Let your journey toward healthy eating be a dance of mindfulness and self-discovery.

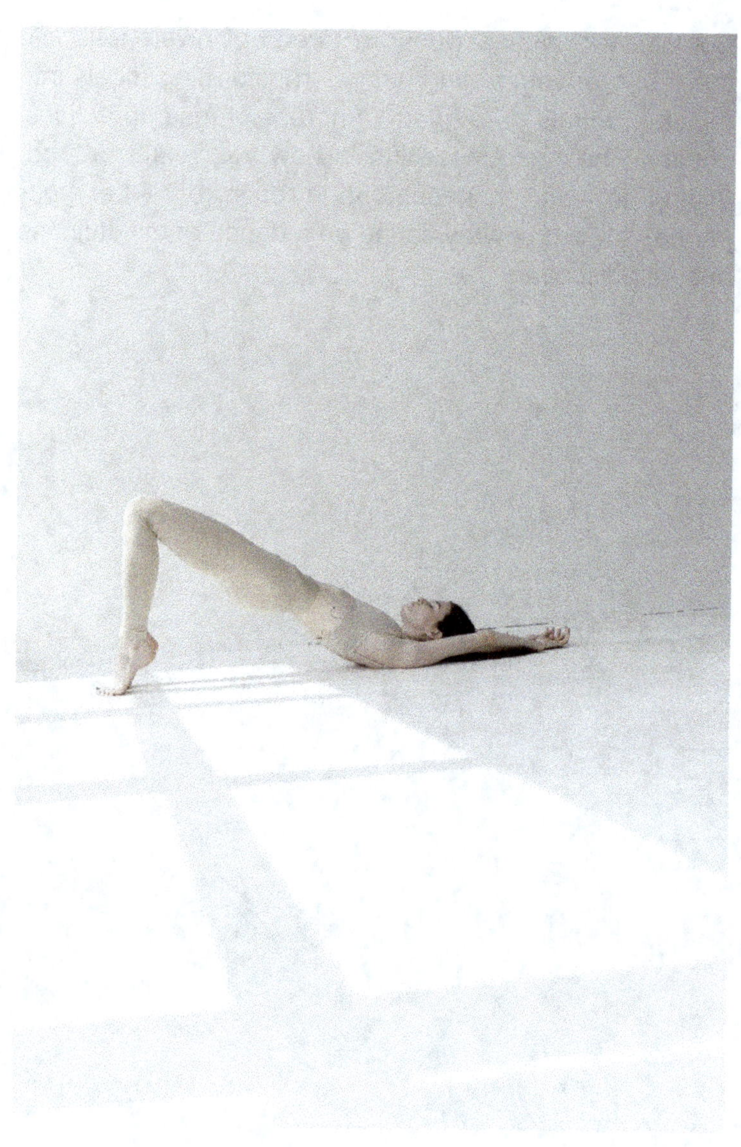

Chapter 6: Crafting Your 30-Day Somatic Exercise Challenge

Setting Realistic Goals

Embarking on a somatic wellness journey involves not just envisioning the destination but also charting a course that is practical, sustainable, and tailored to your unique needs. Let's explore the art of setting realistic goals—milestones that become stepping stones towards a healthier, more connected you.

1. Understanding Your Starting Point:

- Begin by understanding your current state of wellness.
- Assess your physical abilities, emotional well-being, and lifestyle factors without judgment.

2. Clarity on What Wellness Means to You:

- Define what wellness means to you personally.
- Consider aspects such as physical fitness, mental health, emotional balance, and overall well-being.

3. Breaking Down Long-Term Goals:

- Long-term goals are essential, but breaking them down is key.

- Divide larger goals into smaller, more manageable steps to make progress more achievable.

4. SMART Goal Setting:

- Utilize the SMART criteria (Specific, Measurable, Achievable, Relevant, Time-bound) for goal setting.
- Make your goals clear, quantifiable, realistic, aligned with your values, and set within a defined timeframe.

5. Prioritizing Self-Care:

- Incorporate self-care into your goals.
- Prioritize habits that nurture your mental and emotional well-being alongside physical health.

6. Setting Realistic Exercise Targets:

- Set exercise goals that align with your current fitness level.
- Gradually increase intensity and duration to avoid burnout or injury.

7. Building Consistency:

- Consistency is key to success.
- Aim for goals that you can sustain over time, forming a foundation for long-term well-being.

8. Adjusting Goals as Needed:

- Be flexible in adjusting your goals.

- Life is dynamic, and your wellness journey should adapt to changing circumstances.

9. Celebrating Small Wins:

- Acknowledge and celebrate small victories.
- Recognizing progress, no matter how modest, reinforces positive habits.

10. Listening to Your Body:

- Tune into your body's signals.
- If a goal feels too ambitious or conflicts with your well-being, be open to adjusting it.

Setting realistic goals is not about aiming low; it's about creating a path that is both challenging and attainable. As you define your wellness goals, envision a journey that respects where you are today and acknowledges the potential for growth. Let each goal be a testament to your commitment to self-care and a celebration of the remarkable journey you are on.

Designing Your Personalized Somatic Exercise Plan

Crafting a somatic exercise plan is like creating a symphony of movements that resonate with your body's needs and aspirations. Let's explore the steps to design a personalized somatic exercise plan that aligns with your wellness goals and celebrates the harmony between your mind and body.

1. Clarifying Your Objectives:

- Begin by clarifying your somatic wellness objectives.
- Identify areas you wish to improve, whether it's flexibility, stress reduction, or enhanced body awareness.

2. Assessing Your Current State:

- Conduct a self-assessment of your current physical state.
- Consider any areas of tension, discomfort, or specific needs that should be addressed.

3. Choosing Somatic Exercises:

- Select somatic exercises that resonate with your objectives.
- Incorporate movements that address your identified areas for improvement.

4. Balancing Movement Types:

- Ensure a balance between different types of movements.
- Include exercises for flexibility, strength, relaxation, and mindful awareness in your plan.

5. Progression and Gradual Intensity:

- Plan for progression in intensity.
- Start with foundational exercises and gradually increase the challenge as your body adapts.

6. Incorporating Mindfulness Practices:

- Integrate mindfulness practices into your routine.
- Mindful breathing, body scans, or meditation can enhance the mind-body connection.

7. Adapting to Your Schedule:

- Tailor your plan to your schedule and lifestyle.
- Choose a frequency and duration of exercise that is realistic and sustainable for you.

8. Addressing Specific Concerns:

- If you have specific physical concerns or health conditions, tailor exercises accordingly.
- Consult with a healthcare professional if needed for personalized guidance.

9. Enjoyable and Engaging Activities:

- Select activities you enjoy.
- When you find joy in your exercises, it becomes easier to maintain consistency.

10. Listening to Your Body:

- Pay attention to how your body responds.
- Modify exercises if needed, and be attuned to signals of comfort or discomfort.

Your personalized somatic exercise plan is a canvas for self-expression and well-being. Embrace the fluidity of your routine, adjusting it as needed to align with your evolving needs. Let each movement be a celebration of the connection between your mind and body, fostering a deeper understanding of your unique self.

Tracking Progress and Adjusting Along the Way

Embarking on a somatic wellness journey is a dynamic process, and your path to well-being is uniquely yours. In this section, we explore the importance of tracking your progress and embracing the flexibility to make adjustments as needed, ensuring your journey remains a fluid and evolving expression of your commitment to self-care.

1. Establishing Baseline Measures:

- Begin by establishing baseline measures for your somatic wellness goals.
- Record details such as flexibility, stress levels, and any specific areas of discomfort or tension.

2. Utilizing Quantifiable Metrics:

- Incorporate quantifiable metrics where applicable.
- Whether it's the duration of your mindfulness practice or the number of repetitions in an exercise, having measurable data aids in tracking progress.

3. Regular Check-Ins:

- Schedule regular check-ins with yourself.
- Reflect on how your body feels, any changes in mood, and overall improvements in your well-being.

4. Keeping a Somatic Journal:

- Maintain a somatic journal.
- Document your experiences, insights, and any observations related to your exercises and mindfulness practices.

5. Photographic or Video Documentation:

- Consider photographic or video documentation.
- Visual evidence can provide a powerful snapshot of your physical progress over time.

6. Embracing Non-Linear Progress:

- Recognize that progress is often non-linear.
- Some days you may feel more flexible or centered than others, and that's completely normal.

7. Listening to Your Body's Feedback:

- Pay attention to your body's feedback.
- If you notice discomfort or tension, use this information to adjust your exercises or practices accordingly.

8. Adjusting Goals as Needed:

- Be open to adjusting your goals.
- Life circumstances, physical conditions, or evolving priorities may warrant modifications to your initial plan.

9. Celebrating Milestones:

- Celebrate milestones, big or small.
- Acknowledge your achievements and the commitment you've shown to your well-being.

10. Seeking Professional Guidance:

- If needed, seek professional guidance.
- A somatic practitioner, physical therapist, or healthcare professional can provide valuable insights and adjustments to your routine.

Your somatic wellness journey is a dynamic exploration of self-discovery. Embrace the process of tracking your progress as a tool for self-awareness and celebrate the small victories along the way. Remember, the ability to make adjustments is a strength, ensuring that your journey remains aligned with your evolving needs and aspirations.

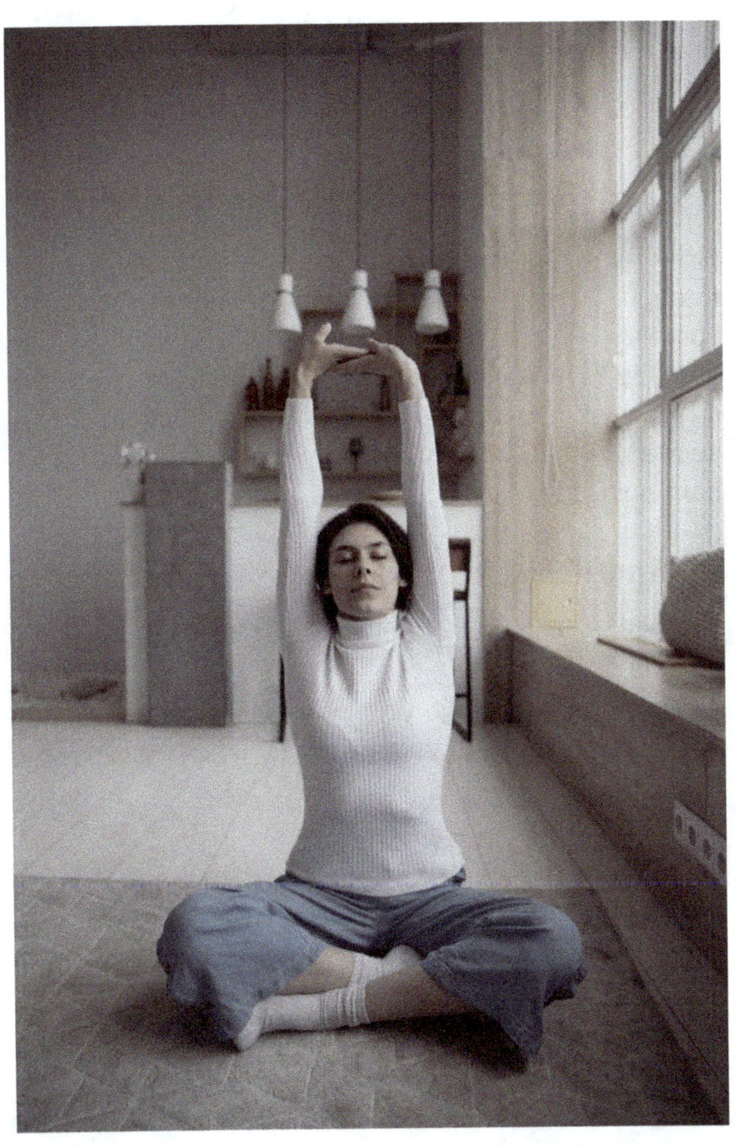

Chapter 7: Daily Routines and Weekly Plans

Morning Wake-Up Somatics

Greet each morning with intention and mindfulness through a rejuvenating session of morning wake-up somatics. This routine is designed to gently awaken your body, enhance flexibility, and cultivate a positive mindset as you embrace the new day. Let's explore a sequence that will invigorate your senses and set a harmonious tone for the hours ahead.

1. Mindful Awakening Breath:

- Begin by lying comfortably on your back or sitting in a relaxed position.
- Inhale deeply through your nose, filling your lungs with air. Exhale slowly through your mouth, releasing any tension.

2. Neck and Shoulder Rolls:

- Slowly roll your shoulders backward and forward.
- Gently turn your head from side to side, feeling the release of tension in your neck.

3. Spinal Twist:

- Sit or stand with a straight spine.
- Slowly twist your upper body to one side, holding for a few breaths. Repeat on the other side.

4. Side Stretches:

- In a standing position, raise one arm overhead and lean gently to the opposite side.
- Feel the stretch along your side. Repeat on the other side.

5. Gentle Forward Bend:

- Stand with your feet hip-width apart.
- Slowly hinge at your hips, allowing your upper body to fold forward. Bend your knees slightly if needed.

6. Hip Circles:

- Stand with feet hip-width apart.
- Circle your hips in a gentle, clockwise motion and then counter-clockwise.

7. Mindful Walking:

- Take a mindful walk, focusing on each step and the connection with the ground.
- Pay attention to the sensations in your feet and legs.

8. Grounding Meditation:

- Find a comfortable seated position.
- Close your eyes and focus on your breath. Visualize roots extending from your body, grounding you to the earth.

9. Arm Swings:

- Stand with your feet shoulder-width apart.
- Swing your arms gently in a circular motion, gradually increasing the size of the circles.

10. Full Body Shake:

- Stand with your feet shoulder-width apart.
- Shake out your arms and legs, letting go of any residual tension.

This morning wake-up somatics routine is your invitation to embrace the day with mindfulness and vitality. Let each movement be a celebration of the present moment, preparing both your body and mind for the opportunities and joys that lie ahead.

Afternoon Energizing Somatic Breaks

Combat the midday fatigue and rejuvenate your body and mind with a series of energizing somatic exercises.

These movements are designed to invigorate your senses, improve circulation, and enhance focus, allowing you to approach the remainder of your day with renewed vitality. Let's embark on a sequence that will uplift your energy levels and provide a refreshing break from the demands of the day.

1. Seated Breath Awareness:

- Find a comfortable seated position.
- Close your eyes and focus on your breath. Inhale deeply through your nose and exhale slowly through your mouth.

2. Shoulder and Neck Release:

- Gently roll your shoulders backward and forward.
- Perform neck stretches by tilting your head to each side and forward, releasing any tension.

3. Dynamic Arm Stretches:

- Stand with your feet hip-width apart.
- Stretch one arm across your chest, holding it with the opposite hand. Switch sides and repeat.

4. Energizing Leg Swings:

- Hold onto a stable surface for support.
- Swing one leg forward and backward, then side to side. Switch legs and repeat.

5. Spinal Twist and Reach:

- Sit or stand with a straight spine.
- Twist your upper body to one side, reaching your arm across. Repeat on the other side.

6. Mindful Walking Break:

- Take a short mindful walk.
- Pay attention to your surroundings and the sensation of movement. Focus on your breath.

7. Somatic Desk Stretch:

- If seated at a desk, perform a seated twist.
- Place one hand on the opposite knee and gently twist your torso, holding for a few breaths. Switch sides.

8. Mindful Breath Reset:

- Pause for a moment of mindful breathing.
- Inhale deeply, fill your lungs, and exhale slowly, releasing any tension.

9. Dynamic Full Body Shake:

- Stand with feet shoulder-width apart.
- Shake out your entire body, letting go of stiffness and fatigue.

10. Grounding Visualization:

- Find a quiet space to sit.

- Close your eyes and visualize yourself connected to the earth, drawing in energy with each breath.

These energizing somatic breaks are your secret weapon against the afternoon slump. Use them to refresh your mind, release tension, and infuse your day with renewed vitality. Let each movement be a mindful break, creating a space for rejuvenation and setting the stage for a productive and energized afternoon.

Evening Relaxation and Stress Release

As the day winds down, give yourself the gift of relaxation and stress release through a series of soothing somatic exercises. These movements are designed to melt away tension, promote a sense of calm, and prepare your body and mind for a restful evening. Let's embark on a journey of gentle movements that invite tranquility and peace into your evening routine.**

1. Gentle Seated Breathing:

- Find a comfortable seated position.
- Inhale deeply through your nose, allowing your abdomen to expand. Exhale slowly through your mouth, releasing any tension.

2. Neck and Shoulder Rolls:

- Sit or stand with a straight spine.
- Gently roll your shoulders backward and forward, releasing tension. Perform gentle neck stretches.

3. Somatic Relaxation Exercises:

- Lie down on your back or find a comfortable reclined position.
- Perform somatic relaxation exercises, focusing on releasing tension from different parts of your body.

4. Mindful Body Scan:

- Close your eyes and bring your attention to your toes.
- Gradually scan your body, releasing tension from each area as you progress upward.

5. Slow Leg Stretch:

- Lie down and extend one leg, flexing and pointing your toes.
- Repeat with the other leg, allowing the stretch to flow through your entire body.

6. Hip Opening Meditation:

- Sit comfortably with a straight spine.
- Focus on your breath and visualize tension leaving your body with each exhale.

7. Somatic Stretches for Lower Back:

- Lie on your back and bring your knees toward your chest.
- Gently rock side to side to release tension in the lower back.

8. Calming Breathwork:

- Practice calming breathwork, such as the 4-7-8 technique.
- Inhale for a count of 4, hold for 7, and exhale for 8.

9. Soothing Leg Up the Wall Pose:

- Sit close to a wall and extend your legs up.
- Relax into the pose, allowing the wall to support your legs.

10. Closing Meditation:

- Sit or lie down comfortably.
- Close your eyes and spend a few minutes in meditation, focusing on gratitude and releasing any remaining stress.

These evening relaxation and stress release exercises are your passport to a tranquil night. Embrace the serenity of these movements, allowing them to guide you into a state of deep relaxation. As you unwind, savor the peace that comes with each breath, letting go of the demands of the day and creating space for a rejuvenating night's rest.

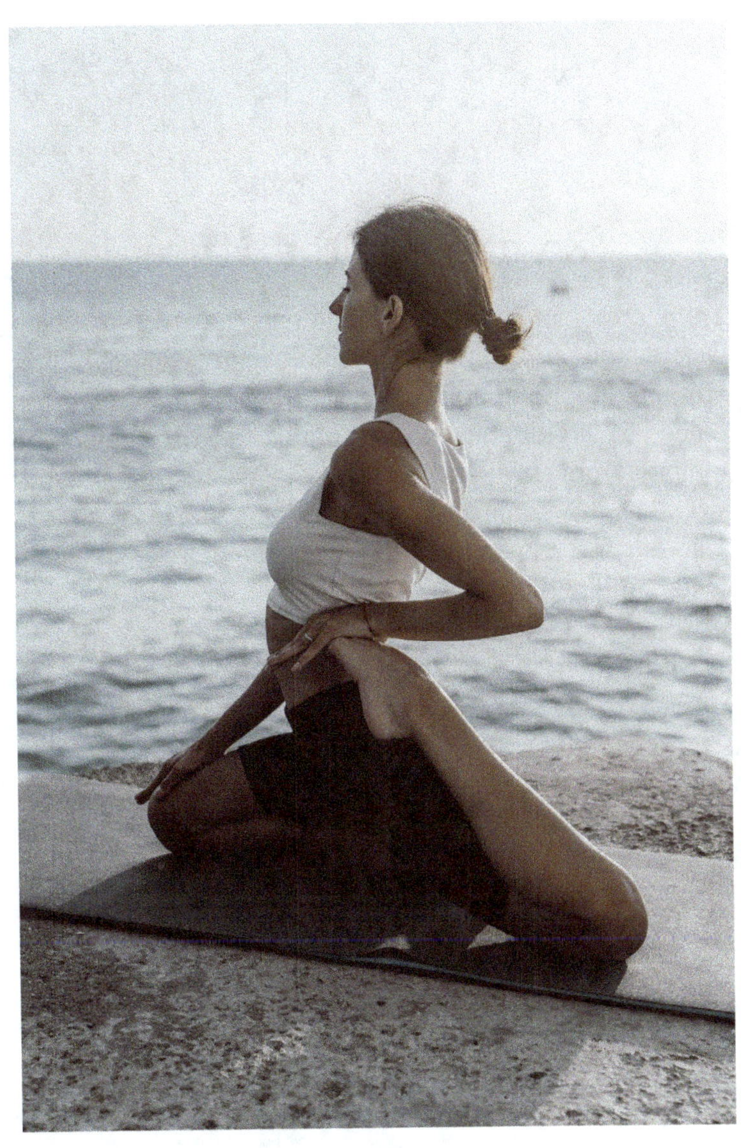

Chapter 8: Integrating Somatics into Daily Life

Somatics at the Office

Transform your workspace into a sanctuary of well-being with simple and effective somatic exercises. Whether you spend long hours at a desk or have a more dynamic office environment, these practices will help you maintain physical and mental vitality throughout your workday. Let's explore a series of somatic exercises tailored for the office setting, promoting relaxation, focus, and overall balance.

1. Seated Mindful Posture Check:

- Sit with your feet flat on the floor and your spine straight.
- Close your eyes and take a moment to mindfully align your posture. Relax your shoulders and breathe deeply.

2. Desk Shoulder Opener:

- Stand or sit and clasp your hands behind your back.
- Gently lift your arms, opening your chest. Hold for a few breaths to release tension in your shoulders.

3. Seated Neck and Upper Back Release:

- Sit comfortably and tilt your head to one side, bringing your ear toward your shoulder.
- Gently release and switch sides. Add a slow head roll for a soothing stretch.

4. Chair Forward Fold:

- Sit forward on your chair with your feet flat on the ground.
- Hinge at your hips and lean forward, reaching for your toes or the floor. Feel the stretch in your lower back and hamstrings.

5. Desk Hip Stretch:

- Sit on the edge of your chair.
- Cross one ankle over the opposite knee, creating a figure-four shape. Lean forward slightly to stretch your hip. Switch sides.

6. Wrist and Hand Release:

- Extend your arms in front of you, palms facing down.
- Gently press down on your fingers with the opposite hand, stretching your wrists. Switch sides.

7. Seated Twist:

- Sit with your feet flat on the floor.

- Twist your torso to one side, placing one hand on the opposite knee. Hold the twist for a few breaths and switch sides.

8. Energizing Desk Leg Lifts:

- Sit with your back straight and lift one leg off the ground.
- Hold for a few seconds, then switch legs. This activates your core and improves circulation.

9. Mindful Breathing Break:

- Take a few minutes for a mindful breathing break.
- Inhale deeply, exhale slowly, and focus on the sensation of your breath to center yourself.

10. Office Walking Meditation:

- Take short mindful walks around the office.
- Focus on each step, bringing awareness to the movement of your body.

Somatics at the office can be a transformative experience, turning your workspace into a haven of well-being. These exercises are your ticket to improved focus, reduced stress, and increased vitality throughout the workday. Embrace these moments of self-care, and let the practice of somatics enhance your work environment with a sense of balance and calm.

Somatic Techniques for Travel

Turn your travel journey into a mindful and rejuvenating experience with simple yet effective somatic techniques. Whether you're on a long flight, a road trip, or navigating through busy airports, these practices are designed to ease tension, promote relaxation, and restore balance to your body and mind. Let's explore a series of somatic techniques tailored for the traveler, ensuring you arrive at your destination with a sense of well-being.

1. Seated Mindful Breathing:

- While seated, close your eyes and take deep, intentional breaths.
- Inhale through your nose, expanding your abdomen, and exhale slowly through your mouth. Repeat to center yourself.

2. Neck and Shoulder Self-Massage:

- Use your fingertips to gently massage your neck and shoulders.
- Release tension by applying circular motions and gradually increasing or decreasing pressure.

3. Seated Spinal Twist:

- Sit with your feet flat on the ground.
- Twist your torso to one side, placing one hand on the opposite knee. Hold for a few breaths, then switch sides.

4. Ankle Rolls and Toe Flexes:

- While seated, roll your ankles in both directions.
- Flex and point your toes to improve circulation and reduce stiffness.

5. Standing Forward Bend:

- Stand with your feet hip-width apart.
- Hinge at your hips and lean forward, allowing your upper body to fold. Release tension in your back and hamstrings.

6. Mindful Walking at the Terminal:

- While navigating through the airport, practice mindful walking.
- Focus on each step, breathing in rhythm with your movement.

7. Seated Cat–Cow Stretch:

- While seated, arch your back and then round it, moving between cat and cow positions.
- This seated variation helps release tension along your spine.

8. Somatic Breathwork for Anxiety:

- If travel induces anxiety, practice somatic breathwork.
- Inhale deeply, hold for a moment, and exhale slowly. Focus on grounding yourself with each breath.

9. Seated Hip Stretch:

- While seated, cross one ankle over the opposite knee.
- Gently press down on the crossed knee to stretch your hip. Switch sides.

10. Mindful Relaxation During Transit:

- During transit, find moments for mindful relaxation.
- Close your eyes, focus on your breath, and visualize a peaceful destination.

Somatic techniques for travel are your companion on the journey, offering moments of self-care amidst the hustle. Embrace these practices to alleviate travel-related tension, connect with your breath, and arrive at your destination with a sense of calm and vitality. Let each movement be a step towards making your travel experience a mindful and rejuvenating adventure.

Incorporating Somatics into Daily Activities

Transform your daily routine into a sanctuary of self-care and mindfulness by seamlessly integrating somatic practices. These simple and effective techniques can be woven into your everyday activities, enhancing your well-being and fostering a deeper mind-body connection. Let's explore how you can infuse the essence of somatics into your daily life, turning each moment into an opportunity for renewal and presence.

1. Morning Mindful Stretching:

- Upon waking, indulge in a mindful stretching routine.
- Reach for the sky, elongate your spine, and gently rotate your wrists and ankles to awaken your body.

2. Mindful Toothbrushing Meditation:

- During your morning and evening toothbrushing, practice mindfulness.
- Focus on the sensations of brushing, the taste of toothpaste, and the gentle movements.

3. Mindful Walking Commute:

- Whether walking to work or during your daily commute, practice mindful walking.
- Pay attention to each step, the rhythm of your breath, and the sights and sounds around you.

4. Desk Chair Mindful Resets:

- Set an hourly reminder to perform a brief somatic reset at your desk.
- Engage in seated stretches, mindful breathing, and subtle movements to release tension.

5. Mindful Eating Rituals:

- Turn your meals into mindful rituals.

- Engage your senses, savor each bite, and take breaks between bites to focus on your breath.

6. Mindful Waiting Moments:

- Turn waiting moments into opportunities for somatic awareness.
- Whether in a line or waiting for an appointment, practice deep breathing and gentle movements.

7. Mindful Phone Use Breaks:

- During phone calls or text responses, take breaks for somatic practices.
- Roll your shoulders, stretch your neck, or simply pause to take a few deep breaths.

8. Mindful Driving Practices:

- Infuse mindfulness into your driving routine.
- Pay attention to your breath, relax your grip on the steering wheel, and be present on the road.

9. Mindful Evening Wind-Down:

- As you wind down in the evening, incorporate mindful stretches and breathwork.
- Release the tensions of the day and transition into a state of relaxation.

10. Mindful Sleep Preparation:

- Establish a mindful sleep routine.

- Practice gentle stretches or a brief body scan before bed to signal your body that it's time for rest.

Incorporating somatics into daily activities is a gentle revolution of self-care. Embrace these practices as invitations to be fully present in each moment, fostering a harmonious connection between your mind and body throughout your day. Let the essence of somatics enrich the ordinary, turning every daily activity into an opportunity for self-renewal and well-being.

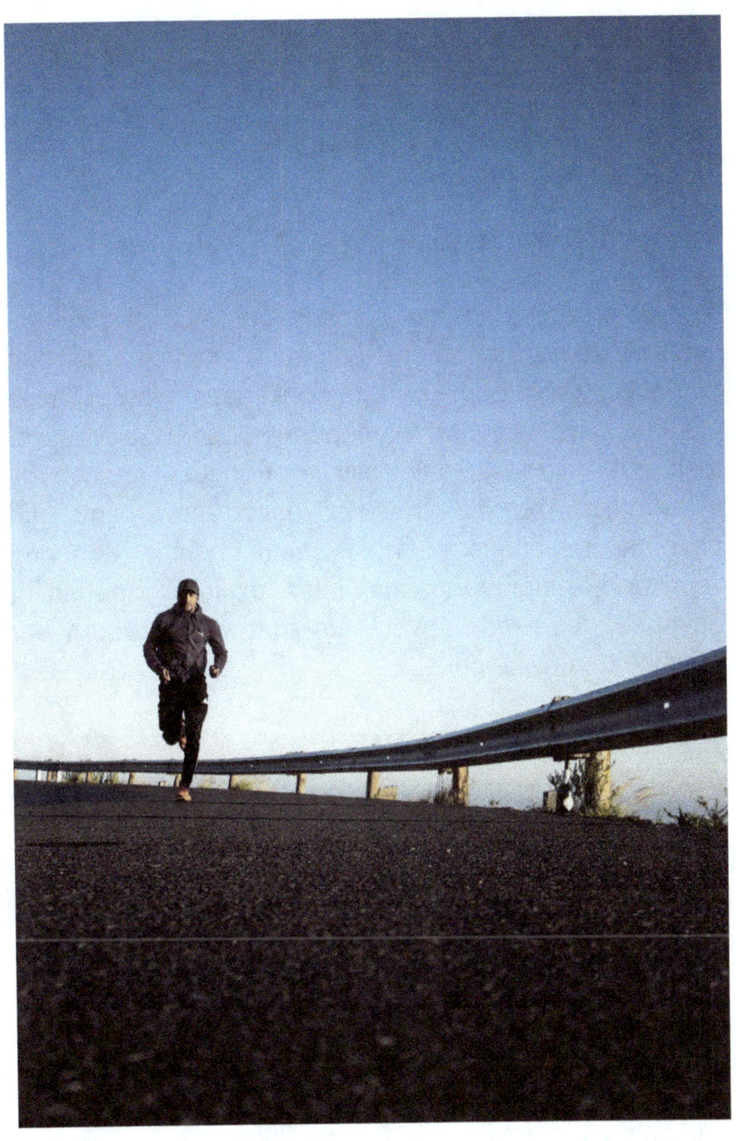

Chapter 9: Enhancing Your Practice

Advanced Somatic Movements

As you progress on your somatic journey, you may find yourself ready for more advanced movements that challenge your body and mind in new ways. These exercises are designed to deepen your somatic practice, fostering increased flexibility, strength, and body awareness. Approach these advanced movements with patience, mindfulness, and a commitment to honoring your body's unique needs. Let's explore a series of advanced somatic movements that will elevate your practice to new heights.

1. Full Body Somatic Wave:

- Stand with feet hip-width apart.
- Initiate a wave-like motion through your body, starting from your feet and traveling up to your head. Reverse the wave back down.

2. Dynamic Hip Circles:

- Stand with feet hip-width apart.
- Perform dynamic hip circles, emphasizing a smooth and controlled movement. Switch directions.

3. Extended Spinal Twist:

- Sit with legs extended.
- Twist your upper body, placing one hand on the opposite knee. Extend your opposite arm behind you for a deeper twist.

4. Somatic Roll-Ups:

- Lie on your back with arms overhead.
- Initiate a somatic roll-up, segmentally rolling through your spine to a seated position. Reverse the movement back down.

5. Balancing Somatic Poses:

- Experiment with advanced balancing poses.
- Examples include one-legged standing poses, such as a somatic tree pose, holding each position mindfully.

6. Somatic Side Plank Variations:

- From a plank position, transition into side plank variations.
- Lift one arm or leg, or experiment with dynamic movements in the side plank position.

7. Dynamic Somatic Lunges:

- Perform dynamic lunges with a somatic twist.
- As you lunge, incorporate a twisting motion, engaging your core and enhancing flexibility.

8. Advanced Somatic Bridge:

- From a supine position, lift into a somatic bridge.
- Experiment with lifting one leg, extending the hips, and engaging your glutes and hamstrings.

9. Flowing Somatic Sequences:

- Create flowing sequences that combine various somatic movements.
- Transition smoothly between exercises, maintaining awareness of your breath and body.

10. Inverted Somatic Poses:

- Explore inverted poses, such as shoulder stands or headstands.
- Approach these poses with caution, ensuring proper alignment and utilizing props if needed.

Advanced somatic movements invite you to explore the edges of your practice, embracing the challenge and growth they offer. As you engage with these movements, prioritize safety, listen to your body, and adapt each exercise to suit your current level of ability. These advanced somatic movements are a testament to the continuous evolution of your practice, bringing new dimensions of strength, flexibility, and mindfulness to your somatic journey.

Somatics for Specific Body Areas

Unlock the potential for deep healing and rejuvenation by focusing on specific areas of your body through targeted somatic movements. These exercises are designed to bring awareness, release tension, and enhance flexibility in key regions. Whether you're looking to strengthen your core, release tension in your hips, or address other specific areas, these somatic movements offer a personalized approach to your well-being. Let's dive into somatics for specific body areas and discover the transformative power of mindful movement.

1. Core Awakening Sequence:

- Start in a seated position and gradually move into a sequence that engages and strengthens the core.
- Include movements like seated twists, somatic roll-ups, and dynamic core contractions.

2. Hip Flexor Release:

- Begin with gentle hip circles in both directions.
- Progress into stretches that focus on releasing tension in the hip flexors, such as lunges and seated hip stretches.

3. Spinal Mobility Flow:

- Develop spinal mobility through a flowing sequence.

- Include cat-cow movements, seated spinal twists, and somatic extensions.

4. Shoulder and Neck Tension Relief:

- Perform somatic movements to release tension in the shoulders and neck.
- Incorporate shoulder rolls, neck stretches, and mindful rotations.

5. Hamstring Flexibility Series:

- Begin with seated hamstring stretches.
- Progress into dynamic movements that improve hamstring flexibility, such as somatic leg swings and seated forward folds.

6. Back Stability and Strength:

- Engage in somatic movements that target the muscles supporting the spine.
- Include somatic bridges, supermans, and other exercises that promote back stability and strength.

7. Somatic Ankle and Foot Mobility:

- Start with ankle circles and toe flexes.
- Move into seated stretches that enhance ankle and foot mobility, fostering better grounding.

8. Mindful Knee Care:

- Practice somatic movements that promote knee stability and flexibility.
- Include gentle knee circles, seated knee extensions, and mindful movements to support knee health.

9. Wrist and Hand Relaxation:

- Address tension in the wrists and hands with somatic stretches.
- Perform circular movements and mindful stretches to release any accumulated stress.

10. Mind-Body Connection Meditation:

- Conclude each session with a mindfulness meditation that connects you with the specific body area you've focused on.
- Visualize the area being bathed in healing energy, fostering a sense of well-being.

Somatics for specific body areas empower you to target and nurture the unique needs of each region. As you engage in these practices, cultivate an attitude of mindfulness and curiosity, paying attention to the sensations and responses of each area. Through the lens of targeted somatic movements, discover the joy of moving with intention and fostering a deeper connection with your body.

Combining Somatics with Other Exercises

Elevate your fitness routine by seamlessly integrating somatic practices with traditional exercises. This synergistic approach enhances the mind-body connection, fostering greater awareness, flexibility, and overall well-being. In this section, we'll explore how you can combine somatic movements with other exercises, creating a dynamic and balanced fitness experience. Let's embark on a journey where the fluidity of somatics meets the strength and conditioning of traditional exercises.

1. Somatic Warm-Up for Cardio Workouts:

- Begin your cardio session with a somatic warm-up.
- Incorporate flowing movements and dynamic stretches to prepare your body for the demands of cardiovascular exercise.

2. Somatic Stretching Between Strength Sets:

- After completing a set of strength exercises, introduce somatic stretches.
- Focus on the muscle groups targeted in the strength exercises to enhance flexibility and reduce post-exercise tension.

3. Mindful Breathing during Yoga Poses:

- Enhance your yoga practice with mindful breathing techniques from somatics.
- During each pose, synchronize your breath with the movements, fostering a deeper mind-body connection.

4. Somatic Cool Down after High-Intensity Workouts:

- Conclude high-intensity workouts with a somatic cool down.
- Engage in gentle movements and stretches to ease your body from an elevated state to a state of relaxation.

5. Somatic Stability Training for Weightlifting:

- Incorporate somatic stability exercises into your weightlifting routine.
- Focus on core-engaging movements to enhance stability during lifts.

6. Somatic Balance Drills in Pilates Sessions:

- Integrate somatic balance exercises into Pilates workouts.
- Challenge your balance through somatic movements, enhancing the effectiveness of Pilates exercises.

7. Somatic Flow within HIIT Workouts:

- Embed somatic flow sequences into high-intensity interval training (HIIT) workouts.
- Enhance the fluidity of your movements while maintaining the intensity of HIIT.

8. Somatic Mindfulness during Mind–Body Classes:

- Infuse somatic mindfulness into mind-body classes like Tai Chi or Qigong.
- Connect with the principles of somatics to deepen your mind-body awareness during these practices.

9. Somatic Mobility Drills for CrossFit Training:

- Integrate somatic mobility drills into your CrossFit routine.
- Improve joint mobility and flexibility to complement the dynamic nature of CrossFit workouts.

10. Somatic Breathwork in Running Sessions:

- Combine somatic breathwork with your running routine.
- Sync your breath with your strides, promoting a rhythmic and mindful running experience.

Combining somatics with other exercises is a transformative approach that harmonizes strength, flexibility, and mindfulness. As you navigate this fusion, listen to your body, and allow the fluidity of somatics to enhance your overall fitness journey. This integrated approach invites you to explore the limitless possibilities of movement, cultivating a balanced and vibrant relationship between your mind and body.

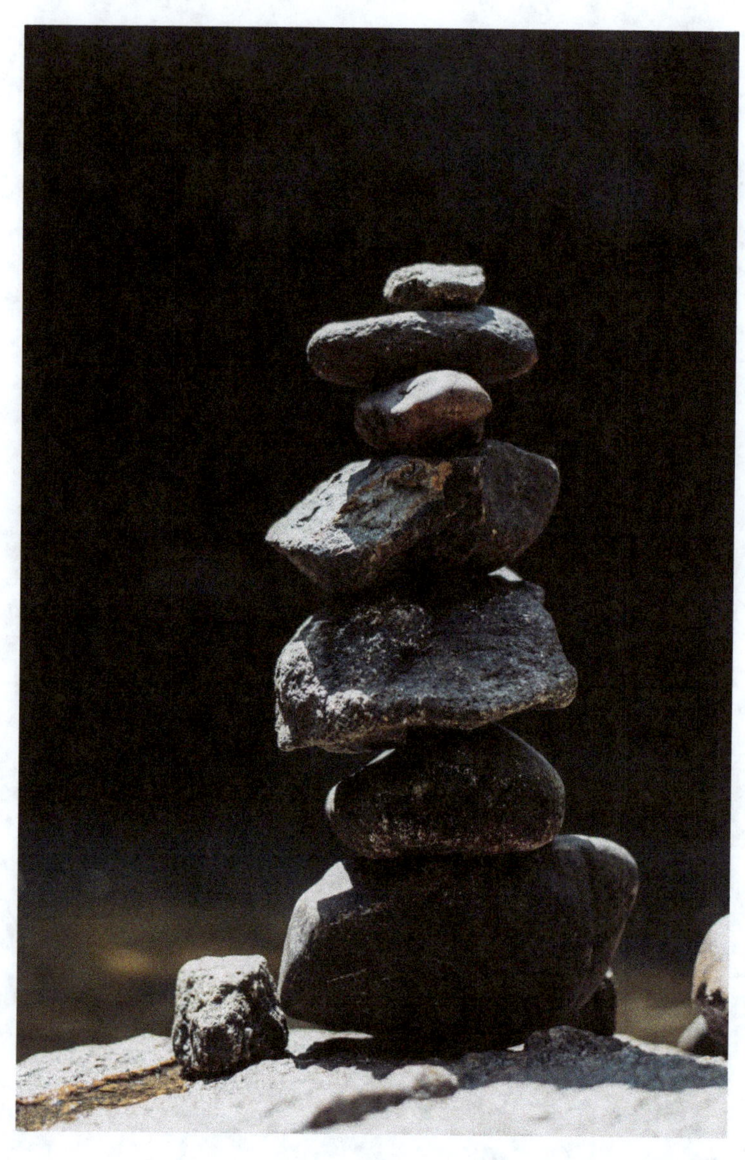

Chapter 10: Holistic Wellness and Somatic Exercise

Somatics Beyond Weight Loss

While somatics is often associated with weight loss, its transformative power extends far beyond the numbers on a scale. In this section, we'll delve into the diverse realms where somatics can profoundly impact your overall well-being. From enhancing mental health to fostering self-awareness, let's explore the myriad ways in which somatics can enrich your life beyond the pursuit of weight loss.

1. Mindful Stress Reduction:

- Engage in somatic practices as a means to reduce stress.
- Use gentle movements, breathwork, and mindfulness to create a sanctuary of calm amidst life's demands.

2. Enhancing Emotional Resilience:

- Explore somatic movements to cultivate emotional resilience.
- Connect with your body's wisdom to navigate and process emotions in a healthy and mindful way.

3. Improving Posture for Confidence:

- Utilize somatic movements to improve posture.
- A strong, aligned posture not only supports physical well-being but also contributes to a sense of confidence and self-assurance.

4. Somatics for Chronic Pain Relief:

- Apply somatic techniques to alleviate chronic pain.
- Mindfully address areas of discomfort, promoting relief and improving your overall quality of life.

5. Boosting Cognitive Function:

- Engage in somatic practices that stimulate cognitive function.
- The mind-body connection nurtured through somatics can enhance memory, focus, and overall mental clarity.

6. Cultivating Body Awareness:

- Use somatic movements to deepen your body awareness.
- This heightened awareness fosters a profound connection with your body, allowing you to respond more intuitively to its needs.

7. Somatics for Better Sleep:

- Develop a somatic bedtime routine for improved sleep.

- Gentle stretches, breathwork, and relaxation techniques can contribute to a restful night's sleep.

8. Mindful Eating Habits:

- Apply somatic principles to cultivate mindful eating.
- Enhance your relationship with food by bringing awareness to each bite and savoring the sensory experience.

9. Somatics for Creativity and Expression:

- Use somatics to unlock creative potential.
- Free your body and mind through expressive somatic movements, fostering a greater connection with your creative spirit.

10. Building Resilience to Life's Challenges:

- Embrace somatics as a tool for building resilience.
- Develop a mindful and adaptable approach to face life's challenges with grace and strength.

Somatics, when embraced beyond weight loss, becomes a holistic practice that touches every facet of your life. From emotional well-being to enhanced cognitive function, the transformative power of somatics extends into realms that contribute to a more vibrant and fulfilling existence. As you explore these dimensions, remember that the journey of somatics is a personal one, uniquely tailored to enrich your life on multiple levels.

Mind-Body Balance and Emotional Well-Being

Harmony between the mind and body is a cornerstone of emotional well-being. In this section, we'll explore how cultivating a balance between your physical and mental realms through somatic practices can lead to a profound sense of emotional harmony. Let's embark on a journey of self-discovery and integration, where the fluid movements of somatics meet the rich landscape of your emotions, fostering a deep sense of well-being.

1. Somatic Grounding Techniques:

- Begin with somatic grounding techniques to anchor yourself in the present moment.
- Engage with the sensations of your body, fostering a sense of stability and calm.

2. Breath-Centric Mindfulness:

- Integrate breath-centric mindfulness with somatic movements.
- Use your breath as a guide, syncing it with your movements to cultivate a centered and peaceful state of mind.

3. Mindful Body Scanning:

- Practice a mindful body scan, systematically bringing awareness to each part of your body.
- This somatic meditation enhances self-awareness and releases tension.

4. Emotional Release Through Movement:

- Use somatic movements as a medium for emotional release.
- Allow your body to express and move through emotions, fostering a sense of liberation.

5. Somatic Yoga for Emotional Balance:

- Combine somatics with yoga poses that promote emotional balance.
- Focus on heart-opening poses and gentle stretches to release emotional tension.

6. Expressive Somatic Arts:

- Engage in expressive somatic arts, such as dance or freeform movement.
- Allow your body to become a canvas for the expression of your emotions.

7. Somatic Relaxation Rituals:

- Develop somatic relaxation rituals for moments of stress.

- Incorporate gentle movements and breathwork to create a sanctuary of calm in your daily life.

8. Mindful Eating for Emotional Nourishment:

- Apply somatic mindfulness to your eating habits.
- Connect with the sensory experience of eating, fostering a healthy relationship with food and emotions.

9. Somatic Practices for Stress Resilience:

- Embrace somatic practices as tools for stress resilience.
- Develop a toolbox of somatic techniques to navigate challenging moments with grace.

10. Cultivating Joy through Movement:

- Infuse joy into your somatic practice.
- Dance, laugh, and move in ways that bring about a sense of joy and lightness.

Mind-body balance is not just a physical state; it's a profound integration of your physical and emotional selves. Through the practice of somatics, you can cultivate a resilient and balanced emotional well-being. As you embark on this journey, remember that each movement is an opportunity to connect with your emotions, fostering a sense of wholeness and vitality.

Building Sustainable Health Habits

Embarking on a journey toward sustainable health habits is a commitment to your well-being that extends far beyond temporary fixes. In this section, we'll explore how somatics can be a guiding force in establishing habits that are not only beneficial for your health but are also enduring and transformative. Let's dive into the principles of building sustainable health habits through mindful movement and intentional living.

1. Setting Realistic and Attainable Goals:

- Begin by setting realistic and attainable health goals.
- Break down larger objectives into smaller, achievable steps, creating a roadmap for success.

2. Consistency over Intensity:

- Prioritize consistency over intensity in your health routine.
- Regular, mindful movements and habits are more sustainable and beneficial in the long run.

3. Integrating Somatic Practices into Daily Rituals:

- Make somatic practices a part of your daily rituals.
- Whether it's morning stretches, midday mindful breaks, or evening relaxation, weave somatics into your routine.

4. Mindful Nutrition Choices:

- Cultivate mindful eating habits.
- Pay attention to what, when, and how you eat, savoring each bite and fostering a healthier relationship with food.

5. Balancing Rest and Activity:

- Achieve balance between rest and activity.
- Listen to your body's cues for rest and engage in somatic movements for active recovery.

6. Stress Management Through Somatics:

- Utilize somatics as a tool for stress management.
- Develop a repertoire of somatic techniques to navigate stress, promoting both mental and physical well-being.

7. Progress Tracking and Celebrating Milestones:

- Track your progress and celebrate milestones, no matter how small.
- Recognize and appreciate the positive changes you're making in your health journey.

8. Community and Accountability:

- Build a supportive community and establish accountability.

- Share your health goals with friends or join groups that align with your objectives, fostering a sense of camaraderie.

9. Adapting to Change:

- Embrace adaptability and be willing to adjust your habits.
- Life is dynamic, and sustainable health habits should be flexible to accommodate change.

10. Cultivating a Positive Mindset:

- Cultivate a positive mindset towards health.
- View your health journey as a lifelong process, focusing on the joy and benefits of the present moment.

Building sustainable health habits is a transformative journey, and somatics can be your steadfast companion. Through intentional, mindful movement and living, you're not just creating habits; you're cultivating a lifestyle that supports your overall well-being. As you integrate somatics into your health routine, remember that the true essence of sustainability lies in the small, consistent choices you make each day.

Chapter 11: Frequently Asked Questions (FAQs)

Common Queries About Somatic Exercise

Navigating the world of somatic exercise may raise questions, and that's perfectly normal. In this section, we'll address some common queries to provide insight, encouragement, and practical guidance as you embark on your somatic journey. Let's dive into the most frequently asked questions about somatic exercise to help you gain a deeper understanding of this transformative practice.

1. What Exactly is Somatic Exercise?

Somatic exercise involves mindful movements and awareness techniques that aim to enhance the connection between the mind and body. It focuses on releasing muscle tension, improving mobility, and fostering a deeper understanding of movement patterns.

2. How is Somatic Exercise Different from Traditional Exercise?

Unlike traditional exercise that often emphasizes external resistance and repetitions, somatic exercise is internal, focusing on the quality of movement, awareness, and releasing muscular tension. It's about retraining the nervous system to move more efficiently.

3. Can Anyone Practice Somatic Exercise?

Absolutely! Somatic exercises are adaptable and can be practiced by individuals of all fitness levels and ages. They are particularly beneficial for those seeking to improve mobility, reduce pain, and enhance overall well-being.

4. Is Somatic Exercise Only for People with Chronic Pain?

While somatic exercise is beneficial for managing chronic pain, it is not limited to those experiencing pain. It is a holistic practice that promotes general well-being, improved posture, increased flexibility, and enhanced mind-body connection.

5. How Soon Can I Expect to See Results?

The timeline for results varies from person to person. Some may experience immediate relief, while others may notice gradual improvements over time. Consistency and mindful practice play a significant role in the effectiveness of somatic exercises.

6. Do I Need Special Equipment for Somatic Exercise?

One of the beauties of somatic exercise is its simplicity. In most cases, you don't need special equipment. Many exercises can be done with just a comfortable mat. Props may occasionally be used to support certain movements.

7. Can Somatic Exercise Help with Stress and Mental Well-Being?

Absolutely. Somatic exercise involves mindful awareness and breathwork, which can significantly contribute to stress reduction and improved mental well-being. The mind-body connection nurtured by somatics promotes a sense of calm and relaxation.

8. How Often Should I Practice Somatic Exercises?

Consistency is key. Starting with a few minutes daily and gradually increasing the duration can be beneficial. Listen to your body, and make somatic exercise a part of your routine that feels sustainable for you.

9. Are Somatic Exercises Suitable for Seniors?

Yes, somatic exercises are gentle and adaptable, making them well-suited for seniors. They can be particularly beneficial for maintaining flexibility, improving balance, and promoting overall mobility in older individuals.

10. Can Somatic Exercise Be Combined with Other Forms of Exercise?

Certainly. Somatic exercise can complement other forms of exercise seamlessly. It can enhance the quality of movement, improve body awareness, and contribute to a more holistic and integrated fitness routine.

Remember, your somatic journey is unique, and these answers serve as general guidance. Feel free to explore and adapt the practice to suit your individual needs and preferences. As you delve into somatic exercise, embrace curiosity and enjoy the transformative journey it offers.

Addressing Concerns and Misconceptions

Embarking on a new approach to wellness, such as somatic exercise, can bring about questions and misconceptions. In this section, we'll address some common concerns and clear up misconceptions to provide you with a comprehensive understanding of somatic exercise. Let's delve into these aspects to ensure you can approach your somatic journey with confidence and clarity.

1. Concern: "Isn't Somatic Exercise Only for People with Chronic Pain?"

While somatic exercise is beneficial for managing chronic pain, it is not exclusive to individuals experiencing pain. Somatics is a holistic practice that enhances overall well-being, improves posture, and fosters a deeper connection between the mind and body.

2. Misconception: "Somatic Exercise Is Just Another Form of Stretching."

Somatic exercise goes beyond traditional stretching. It involves mindful movements and awareness techniques designed to release chronic muscle tension by reprogramming the nervous system. It's about quality of movement, not just reaching a particular stretch.

3. Concern: "Will Somatic Exercise Make Me More Flexible, But Weaker?"

Quite the opposite. Somatic exercise aims for a balanced approach. By releasing unnecessary muscle tension, somatics can enhance flexibility without sacrificing strength. It's about optimizing the functioning of muscles, promoting both flexibility and strength.

4. Misconception: "Somatic Exercise Takes a Long Time to See Results."

Results can vary, but many people experience immediate improvements. Consistency is key. Regular, mindful practice enhances the effectiveness of somatic exercise. Gradual, sustained changes often lead to lasting benefits.

5. Concern: "Do I Need to Be Flexible or Fit to Start Somatic Exercise?"

Not at all. Somatic exercises are adaptable to all fitness levels. They are accessible to beginners and can be tailored to suit individual needs. Somatics is about meeting your body where it is and gently progressing from there.

6. Misconception: "Somatic Exercise Is Only About Relaxation."

While relaxation is one aspect, somatic exercise is comprehensive. It includes mindful movements, breathwork, and awareness techniques that can be both calming and invigorating. The focus is on holistic well-being.

7. Concern: "Can Somatic Exercise Be Done by Seniors?"

Absolutely. Somatic exercises are gentle and adaptable, making them well-suited for seniors. They can be particularly beneficial for maintaining flexibility, improving balance, and promoting overall mobility in older individuals.

8. Misconception: "I Need Special Equipment for Somatic Exercise."

Somatic exercise is often equipment-free. While props might be occasionally used, many exercises can be done with just a comfortable mat. Simplicity is a key feature of somatics.

9. Concern: "Will Somatic Exercise Make My Muscles Weaker?"

No, it won't. Somatic exercise seeks to optimize muscle function, releasing unnecessary tension. By doing so, it often enhances both flexibility and strength, contributing to overall muscle health.

10. Misconception: "Somatic Exercise Is Only for Mindful People."

Somatic exercise can be enjoyed by anyone, regardless of their familiarity with mindfulness. The practice itself cultivates mindfulness, and you can gradually incorporate this aspect into your routine.

Remember, your somatic journey is personal, and these responses serve as general guidance. As you delve into somatic exercise, feel free to embrace your own experiences, and if any concerns arise, don't hesitate to explore and seek guidance. Your somatic journey is a unique path, and the practice is designed to be adaptable to your individual needs.

Chapter 12: Celebrating Your Somatic Journey

Reflecting on Your Progress

As you engage in the practice of somatic exercise, taking moments to reflect on your journey can deepen your understanding, celebrate achievements, and guide your next steps. In this section, we'll explore the significance of reflection in the context of somatic exercise and provide you with prompts and insights to enhance your introspective practice. Let's embark on a mindful journey of self-discovery and progress.

1. Recognizing Physical Changes:

Take note of any shifts in your physical well-being. Are you experiencing increased flexibility, reduced tension, or improved posture? Reflect on how these changes contribute to your overall comfort and movement.

2. Understanding Emotional Resilience:

Consider how your emotional landscape has evolved. Have you noticed an increased ability to manage stress or a greater sense of emotional resilience? Reflect on the emotional benefits you've gained through somatic practice.

3. Exploring Mind-Body Connection:

Delve into your mind-body connection. How has your awareness of movement patterns and sensations evolved? Reflect on moments where you felt a deep connection between your physical and mental states.

4. Celebrating Small Achievements:

Celebrate small victories along the way. Reflect on the milestones you've achieved, whether it's holding a pose with more ease, maintaining mindful breathing, or integrating somatic exercises into your daily routine.

5. Adapting to Challenges:

Consider how you've navigated challenges. Reflect on your ability to adapt and learn from setbacks. Acknowledge the lessons you've gained from moments of difficulty.

6. Enhancing Mindfulness in Daily Life:

Examine how mindfulness has seeped into your daily life. Reflect on moments where you've applied somatic principles outside your practice, such as being present in daily activities or making mindful choices.

7. Setting New Intentions:

As you reflect on your journey, consider if your intentions have shifted. Are there new aspects of somatic exercise you want to explore? Reflect on how your goals and aspirations are evolving.

8. Noticing the Unseen:

Look beyond the obvious. Reflect on subtle changes that might not be immediately apparent. These could be shifts in your mindset, increased self-awareness, or a more positive relationship with your body.

9. Sharing Your Journey:

Reflect on the idea of sharing your somatic journey. Whether with a friend, a community, or through journaling, consider how expressing your experiences can enhance your connection to the practice.

10. Gratitude for the Journey:

Express gratitude for your somatic journey. Reflect on the privilege of taking this transformative path and appreciate the growth, self-discovery, and well-being it has brought into your life.

Reflection is a powerful tool in your somatic toolkit. As you embark on this journey, let each reflection be a moment of self-discovery and affirmation. Your progress is unique and personal, and this introspective practice is a vital companion on your path to holistic well-being.

Embracing the New You

As you progress through the practice of somatic exercise, you are not only cultivating physical changes but also nurturing a deeper connection with yourself. In this section, let's explore the transformative journey you've embarked on and how you can wholeheartedly embrace the new you that is emerging through mindful movement and self-awareness.

1. Acknowledging Personal Growth:

Take a moment to acknowledge your personal growth. How have you evolved since the beginning of your somatic journey? Recognize the strengths, resilience, and newfound wisdom that have emerged.

2. Cultivating Self-Compassion:

Extend compassion to yourself. Embrace the learning curve and acknowledge that growth comes with both challenges and triumphs. Cultivate a nurturing inner dialogue that supports your evolving self.

3. Celebrating Body Appreciation:

Celebrate your body as it is right now. Reflect on the ways in which your body serves you. Appreciate its resilience, its ability to move, and the positive changes you've experienced.

4. Mindful Presence in the Moment:

Embrace the present moment with mindfulness. Allow yourself to fully inhabit the now, appreciating the journey you're on. Mindful presence fosters a deeper connection with yourself and your surroundings.

5. Expressing Gratitude for Your Body:

Express gratitude for your body. Reflect on the gratitude you feel for the support, movement, and sensations your body provides. Embracing gratitude enhances the positive connection with your physical self.

6. Embracing Self-Discovery:

Acknowledge the ongoing process of self-discovery. Reflect on the aspects of yourself that you've uncovered or rediscovered through somatic exercise. Embracing self-discovery is a continual, enriching journey.

7. Letting Go of Judgment:

Release self-judgment. Embrace the new you without attaching judgment to your journey. Every step is a valuable part of your growth. Let go of unrealistic expectations and embrace the authenticity of your path.

8. Connecting with Joyful Movement:

Engage in joyful movement. Embrace the sheer joy of moving your body. Whether it's dancing, stretching, or simply enjoying the sensation of breath, let joy be a guiding force in your somatic practice.

9. Affirming Your Worthiness:

Affirm your worthiness. Reflect on the inherent value you possess as a unique individual. Embrace the understanding that you are worthy of love, care, and the investment in your well-being.

10. Carrying the Lessons Forward:

Consider how you can carry the lessons learned in your somatic practice into other aspects of your life. Embrace the integration of mindfulness, self-compassion, and body awareness in your daily experiences.

Embracing the new you is a journey of self-love, acceptance, and continual growth. As you immerse yourself in the transformative practice of somatic exercise, remember that you are not only reshaping your body but also fostering a profound connection with your true self. Celebrate the emerging you, and let this journey be a testament to the beauty of your ongoing evolution.

Building a Lifelong Somatic Practice

Embarking on a lifelong somatic practice is a commitment to your holistic well-being. In this section, we'll explore the principles and habits that can help you not only integrate somatic exercise into your daily life but also foster a lifelong journey of mindful movement and self-discovery. Let's delve into the foundations of building a sustainable and enriching somatic practice.

1. Making It a Daily Ritual:

Make somatic exercise a part of your daily ritual. Whether it's a morning stretch, a midday mindful break, or an evening relaxation routine, consistent daily practice reinforces the mind-body connection.

2. Adapting to Your Schedule:

Adapt somatic exercises to fit your schedule. Recognize that life is dynamic, and your practice can be flexible. Short, focused sessions can be just as beneficial as longer ones.

3. Exploring Various Somatic Modalities:

Explore different somatic modalities. From yoga-inspired movements to Feldenkrais techniques, diversity in your practice adds richness and keeps your routine engaging.

4. Combining Somatics with Other Activities:

Integrate somatic principles into other activities. Whether you're walking, gardening, or sitting at your desk, infusing somatic awareness into daily activities enhances mindfulness and promotes continuous learning.

5. Listening to Your Body:

Cultivate a habit of listening to your body. Regularly check in with how you feel physically and emotionally. Adjust your practice based on your body's signals, fostering a harmonious relationship.

6. Setting Realistic Goals:

Set realistic and achievable goals. Recognize that progress in somatic practice is often gradual. Celebrate small victories, and let your goals evolve with your growing understanding of your body.

7. Continuing Education:

Engage in ongoing learning. Attend workshops, read books, and explore online resources to deepen your understanding of somatic exercise. Lifelong learning keeps your practice vibrant and evolving.

8. Creating a Sacred Space:

Designate a sacred space for your practice. Whether it's a corner of a room or a peaceful outdoor spot, having a dedicated space enhances the ritualistic aspect of your somatic practice.

9. Building a Community:

Connect with a somatic community. Share experiences, insights, and challenges with others on a similar journey. A supportive community can provide inspiration and motivation.

10. Teaching and Sharing:

Consider teaching or sharing somatic practices with others. Whether informally with friends or family or more formally in a class setting, sharing your knowledge deepens your understanding and enriches your practice.

Building a lifelong somatic practice is about weaving mindful movement into the fabric of your life. It's not just about exercises; it's a journey of self-discovery, well-being, and continual growth. As you commit to this transformative practice, let it be a source of joy, resilience, and a lifelong exploration of the incredible connection between your mind and body.

Conclusion

Your Ongoing Somatic Adventure

Welcome to the ever-evolving journey of somatic exploration! In this section, we'll embrace the spirit of adventure as we navigate the continuous terrain of somatic practice. This is not a destination; it's a dynamic and enriching adventure that unfolds with every breath and movement. Let's delve into the heart of your ongoing somatic adventure.

1. Embracing Curiosity:

Cultivate an attitude of curiosity. Approach each somatic session with a sense of wonder, eager to explore new movements, sensations, and insights. The adventure lies in the discoveries along the way.

2. Mindful Movement Exploration:

View your somatic practice as a playground of mindful movement. Experiment with variations, modifications, and different speeds. Allow your body to express itself in a way that feels natural and liberating.

3. Celebrating Uniqueness:

Celebrate your unique journey. Your body is unlike any other, and your somatic adventure is uniquely yours.

Revel in the beauty of your individuality and the discoveries that only you can make.

4. Riding the Waves of Change:

Acknowledge that your somatic adventure will have peaks and valleys. Like any journey, there will be moments of exhilaration and challenges. Embrace the undulating rhythm, knowing that each wave carries valuable lessons.

5. Connecting with Breath as a Guide:

Let your breath be your guide through this adventure. Explore how different breathing patterns influence your movements and sensations. Your breath is a constant companion, guiding you through the landscapes of your body.

6. Finding Joy in Movement:

Seek joy in your movements. Whether it's a gentle stretch, a flowing sequence, or a moment of stillness, infuse joy into your practice. The adventure becomes even more fulfilling when joy is your companion.

7. Nurturing Self–Compassion:

Extend compassion to yourself on this adventure. There are no judgments or destination points; there's only the unfolding present. Let self-compassion be the gentle breeze that propels you forward.

8. Dancing with Challenges:

Dance with challenges rather than resisting them. Challenges are not roadblocks but invitations for growth. Your ability to adapt and learn becomes a dance that enhances the richness of your somatic adventure.

9. Weaving Somatic Wisdom into Daily Life:

Extend your somatic adventure beyond your practice mat. Weave somatic principles into your daily life. Feel the grace in your step, the alignment in your posture, and the mindfulness in your breath as you navigate the world.

10. Savoring the Present Moment:

Savor the richness of the present moment. Your ongoing somatic adventure is happening now. It's not about reaching a destination but reveling in the beauty of each step, each breath, and each sensation.

Your somatic adventure is a canvas waiting to be painted with the brushstrokes of your movements, breath, and awareness. As you navigate this ongoing exploration, relish the excitement of the unknown, the beauty of self-discovery, and the joy of living in harmony with your body. Welcome to the endless adventure of somatic practice!

Recommendation

As you conclude your transformative journey through "Somatic Exercise for Weight loss," consider diving deeper into the world of mindful movement with "Wall Pilates for weight Loss: Wall to Wellness for Women." Authored by myself, this book is a comprehensive guide to integrating Pilates principles with the support of a wall.

Why Wall Pilates?

1. **Efficient Core Activation:** Explore a unique approach to core activation using the stability of the wall. Wall Pilates engages your core muscles effectively, fostering strength and stability from the inside out.*

2. **Enhanced Flexibility:** Discover how the wall can be a versatile tool for improving flexibility. The exercises in this book guide you through dynamic movements that enhance your range of motion.

3. **Mindful Alignment:** Build a heightened awareness of your body's alignment with Wall Pilates. The wall becomes a guide, helping you maintain proper form and posture throughout each movement.

4. **Accessible Home Workouts:** Whether you're a seasoned Pilates enthusiast or a beginner, the wall provides a stable support for various exercises. Enjoy effective Pilates workouts in the comfort of your home.

5. **Incorporating Props:** Explore how simple props, combined with the support of the wall, can add versatility to your Pilates routine. From resistance bands to stability balls, discover creative ways to enhance your practice & more.

www.ingramcontent.com/pod-product-compliance
Lightning Source LLC
Chambersburg PA
CBHW050824260726
48660CB00004B/1587